Radiation Therapy

Edited by Thomas J. FitzGerald

Published in London, United Kingdom

Radiation Therapy
http://dx.doi.org/10.5772/intechopen.104154
Edited by Thomas J. FitzGerald

Contributors
Jozef Sabol, Eter Natelauri, Jonathan B. Wallach, Chana Stern, Michael Karp, David L. Schwartz, Katsiaryna Hancharova, Anatoly Batyan, Pavel Dziameshka, Viktar Lemiasheuski, Aliaksandr Orgish, Paula Elaine Diniz dos Reis, Beatriz Regina Lima de Aguiar, Eliete Neves Silva Guerra, John A. Kalapurakal, Samir Patel, Andrea Lo, Luke E. Pater, Mary Frances McAleer, Arnold Paulino, Carolina de la Pinta

First published in London, United Kingdom, 2023 by IntechOpen
IntechOpen is the global imprint of INTECHOPEN LIMITED, registered in England and Wales, registration number: 11086078, 5 Princes Gate Court, London, SW7 2QJ, United Kingdom

British Library Cataloguing-in-Publication Data
A catalogue record for this book is available from the British Library

Additional hard and PDF copies can be obtained from orders@intechopen.com

Radiation Therapy
Edited by Thomas J. FitzGerald
p. cm.
Print ISBN 978-1-80355-933-9
Online ISBN 978-1-80355-934-6
eBook (PDF) ISBN 978-1-80355-935-3

For EU product safety concerns:
IN TECH d.o.o., Prolaz Marije Krucifikse Kozulić 3, 51000 Rijeka, Croatia,
info@intechopen.com or visit our website at intechopen.com.

Meet the editor

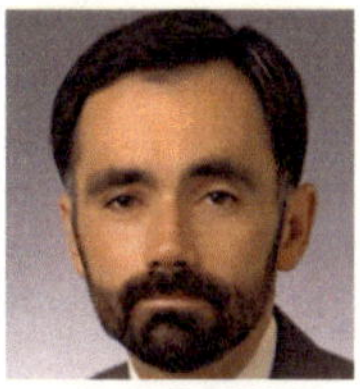

Dr. Thomas J. FitzGerald is a professor and chair of the Department of Radiation Oncology, University of Massachusetts Medical School, USA. He is one of the primary investigators of the Imaging and Radiation Oncology Core (IROC) and directs the Quality Assurance Review Center (QARC), which provides quality assurance and data management for the National Clinical Trials Network (NCTN) and industry trials. His area of clinical expertise is in the application of advanced technology radiation therapy into patient care coupled with a longstanding basic science interest in bone marrow radiobiology and cellular adhesion molecules that serve as biomarkers for therapeutic resistance.

Contents

Preface

This book offers a comprehensive review of challenges and opportunities in the modern application of radiation therapy. As therapy has evolved into calculating radiation dose as a volume and applying modern tools for treatment execution, this book addresses several issues that affect modern management. Dose modeling processes are evolving into three- and four-dimensional processes and this book examines how linear quadratic models can be repurposed for treatment execution and computation. This will be especially important as additional layers of care including brachytherapy and radiopharmaceutical care become commonplace and part of daily composite radiation therapy treatment planning integrating the role of radiation therapy dose rate and radiobiological effectiveness with different therapy treatment modalities. Multiple image sets will be required for fusion into radiation therapy planning imaging in order to generate target volumes for treatment. The role of radiogenomics and dose painting will expand to include dose augmentation to volumetric subsets of tumor areas representing features consistent with both resistance and response to therapy. Modern aspects of care for patients with cervical cancer, prostate cancer, and hepatic therapy are discussed at length and represent many of the challenges of modern care. Finally, the last chapter helps define the ultimate goal of our practice by defining the late effects of treatment and what we should consider to mitigate these issues for patients moving forward. We wish to thank all the contributing authors and we hope you enjoy the book.

Thomas J. FitzGerald MD
Department of Radiation Oncology,
University of Massachusetts Medical School,
Worcester, MA, USA

Chapter 1

Basic Radiation Protection for the Safe Use of Radiation and Nuclear Technologies

Jozef Sabol

Abstract

Any use of both ionizing radiation and nuclear technologies requires ensuring appropriate safety and security of persons as well as the adequate protection of the environment. This is why the applications and handling of sources of ionizing radiation should be in line with the relevant national and international standards containing appropriate safety and security requirements and recommendations. In order to understand and follow these standards, it is necessary to assess the related radiation risks, which should be quantified by using specific dosimetry and radiation protection quantities and units. The chapter introduces and discusses these quantities and units aimed at the evaluation of the biological harms attributed to both stochastic and deterministic effects. The correct use and interpretation of radiation quantities are important to follow relevant regulations and to communicate radiation risks to workers and the public. The chapter takes into account the latest situation in the field, relying on the recent position of relevant international expert bodies.

Keywords: radiation, protection, use of radiation, radiation technologies, international standards

1. Introduction

Radiation can be divided into two groups, namely *ionizing radiation* and *nonionizing radiation*. While ionizing radiation of sufficient energy is able to ionize the atoms of the matter with which it interacts, nonionizing radiation has not this ability. In general, **ionizing radiation**—particles or electromagnetic waves—carries enough energy to knock electrons from atoms or molecules, thereby ionizing them. The result is a positive ion and a free electron, which may be later attached to a neutral atom, thus forming a negative ion.

An illustration of nonionizing and ionizing radiation wavelengths (from the left with increasing values to the right) is shown in **Figure 1** (based on [1]).

In principle, ionizing radiation can be directly ionizing radiation (charged particles) and indirectly ionizing radiation represented by photons (gamma, X-ray, annihilation photons) and neutrons. The interaction of this radiation can also result in

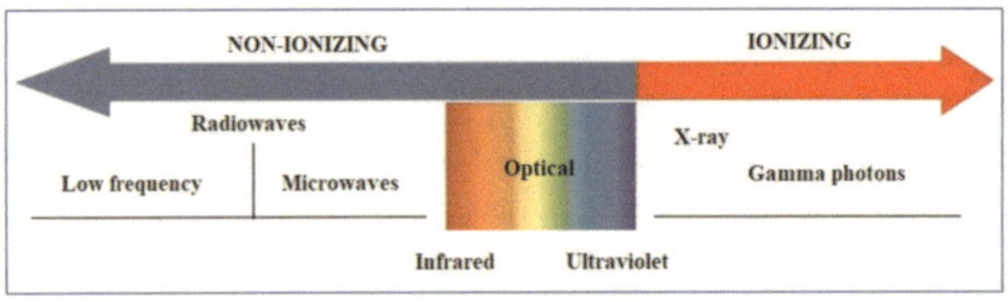

Figure 1.
Nonionizing and ionizing photon radiation.

positive and negative ions and free electrons, which were created by secondary charged particles released by the interaction of indirectly ionizing radiation with matter. It means that indirectly ionizing radiation is ionizing the matter through the charged particles released by such interactions as photoeffect, Compton effect, and pair production. Neutrons themselves cannot directly ionize atoms. They do it through charged particles released as a result of their interaction with matter.

This chapter will deal *only with ionizing radiation* (further only as radiation). As to its interaction with matter, the following processes should be considered:

- Interaction of charged particles such as electrons, protons, alpha particles, and heavy ions;
- Interaction of electromagnetic radiation causing the removal of one of the orbital electrons accompanying by the bremsstrahlung (braking radiation) and production of characteristic radiation;
- Neutron interaction includes a variety of processes characterized by elastic and inelastic scattering and other nuclear reactions, which may lead to the initiation of both charged and uncharged particles.

Radiation is emitted by sources, which may be in the principle of two categories: *radioactive sources* and *radiation generators*. Radioactive sources (radionuclides) produce radiation that produces, as a result of the decay of unstable nuclei, radiation continuously, and the process cannot be stopped. Radiation generators (X-ray tubes and charged particle accelerators) produce radiation only when appropriate conditions are created. This requires a power supply from outside. When the supply is disconnected or switched off, the production of radiation will be stopped.

These features of two different radiation sources have a significant implication for radiation protection. On one side, we have sources that continuously emit radiation whether we use them, transport or store them, and we have to keep them under control all the time. As to radiation generators, the care for radiation protection is much simpler since when they are not in operation practically, no protection measures should be in place.

For safety reasons, it is important to use standard warning signs in places where radioactive sources, radioactive or nuclear waste, and radiation generators are present (**Figure 2**).

The term radiation protection is used universally with the meaning of radiation safety or radiation security. Strictly speaking, one may apply these terms in a more specific manner: radiation safety is related to ensuring people and the environment

Figure 2.
Radiation warning signs, a) a universal sign, b) a new symbol of radiation presence (based on [2, 3]).

against harmful effects of radiation emitted by the source, while radiation (nuclear) security is associated with providing sufficient protection of the source of radiation against a person who may not be aware of the source or who may use it to commit a malevolent or terrorist attack.

2. Biological effects of radiation exposure

It is well-known fact that radiation can be harmful to the human body. Biological and medical knowledge about the effects of ionizing radiation has been gained since the beginning of the last century and is currently extensive but not yet complete. They include observations of clinical, experimental, and above all, group investigations, which are necessary to demonstrate an increased frequency of those diseases that are clinically indistinguishable from spontaneous diseases (e.g., cancer).

The health effects caused by radiation exposure fall into two groups: stochastic effects and deterministic effects (tissue reactions).

The *stochastic effects* of radiation are those effects that we do not know with certainty that they will manifest after exposure; they are manifested only with a certain probability. This includes an increased risk of cancer and hereditary diseases. On the other hand, deterministic effects appear only above a certain level of exposure (dose), which is relatively high. In both cases, the effects may affect a person exposed (somatic effects) or his offspring (genetic effects), as shown in **Figure 3**.

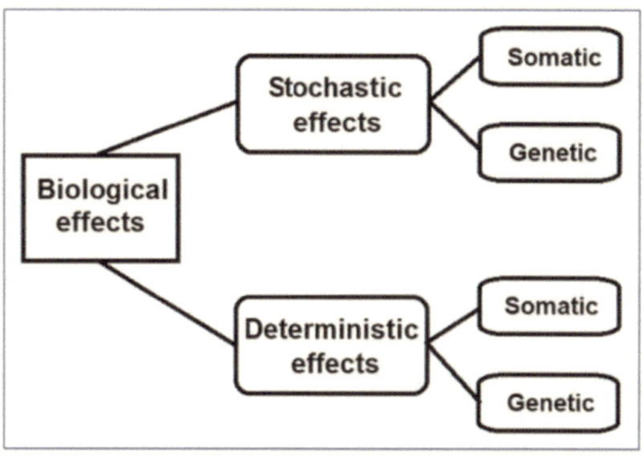

Figure 3.
An overview of the biological effects of radiation on the person and their offspring.

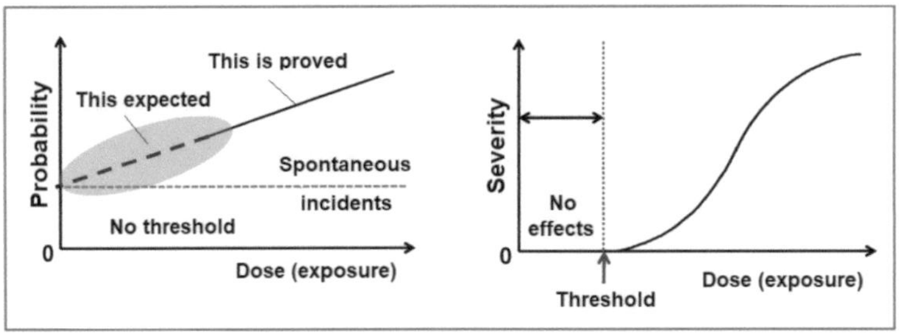

Figure 4.
Comparison between stochastic and deterministic effects.

The *stochastic effects* are caused by the mutations (changes in the genetic information of the cell) and are characterized by a threshold-free, linear dose-response relationship. The dose dependence of these effects is statistical in nature, and therefore, the designation stochastic effects (probable, accidental) have been introduced for them. The size of the radiation dose does not change the severity of the individual's manifestation, but in the population, it changes the frequency of the additional appearance of malignant neoplasms and hereditary damage. Thus, with the dose, the likelihood of injury increases for the individual.

The exposure above certain threshold results in deterministic effects where the severity of the body reaction is roughly proportional to the exposure (**Figure 4**). Exposure to radiation under this level causes no impact.

3. Quantification of stochastic and deterministic effects

The interaction of radiation with matter leads to the deposition of some or full of its energy in the absorption medium, the temperature of which may increase. Since the deposition energy is very low, this is not the main cause of consequent effects in the living tissues where the type of particles, the density of the energy lost per unit of the tracking sensitivity of different tissues exposed, and other factors play a more significant role. This is why the response of the body cannot be expressed by pure physical quantities, and other factors related to the tissue reactions to formed radicals are of primary importance.

The risk created by radiation to the human body cannot be expressed by means of only physical quantities and some specific quantities—we may call them *biophysical* rather than *physical quantities.* The biophysical quantities are based on the physical quantities weighted by specific factors taking into account the biological harm of various types of radiation as well as the sensitivity of particular organs and tissues to the exposure.

3.1 Physical quantities and units

One of the first attempts to quantify radiation exposure to a person was based on ionizing abilities of radiation (at that time, only X-ray photos were assumed) where a unit *roentgen* was introduced as a measure of the ability of photons to ionize the air. Later on, the roentgen (R) became a unit of a quantity *exposure*, introduced by the equation

$$X = \frac{dQ}{dm} \tag{1}$$

where dQ is the total charge of the ions of one sign generated by the electrons (negatrons and positrons) produced by photons in the mass of air dm.

The SI unit of this quantity is C kg^{-1}, the relation with the old unit—roentgen (R)—is 1 R = 2.58 × 10^{-4} C.kg^{-1} (exactly). Because of the definitions, the quantity of exposure could be applied in practice only to photons of energy up to about 300 keV [4].

Later on, when radiation protection had to address the results of interactions of other types of radiations, including beta, alpha, neutrons, and others, a universal quantity of (absorbed) dose was introduced. This is a universal physical quantity reflecting the deposition of radiation in any substance. The *dose* was introduced as follows:

$$D = \frac{dE_i}{dm} \tag{2}$$

where dE_i is the mean energy imparted to the matter of mass dm. The unit of the dose and the dose rate are Gy (gray) and Gy.h^{-1} (gray per hour). Commonly, units mGy, μGy, and mGy h^{-1} or μGy.h^{-1} are frequently used. Before, for the old unit, the rad unit was in use, where 1 Gy = 100 rad [5].

The dose is considered to be a universal quantity in dosimetry, and it is a basis for most quantities used in radiation protection. It can be used for any type of radiation and for any medium or absorber.

The last physical quantity to be mentioned here is the *kerma (K)*, which is the acronym for Kinetic Energy Released per unit Mass. This quantity can only be used for photons and neutrons in any media. It is still widely used especially in computational dosimetry. The kerma is defined by the equation

$$K = \frac{dE_{tr}}{dm} \tag{3}$$

where dE_{tr} is the sum of the initial kinetic energies of all the charged particles liberated by uncharged particles in a mass dm of material. The medium should always be specified.

The special name for the unit of kerma is gray (Gy); the unit for the kerma and dose is thus the same. In addition, here, one can specify this quantity related to the unit of time as the *kerma rate*, defined as the kerma per second. The main unit for this quantity is analogical to the dose rate, i.e., Gy.s^{-1}.

The illustration of the dose and kerma is shown in **Figure 5**, documenting their relationship. It is obvious that the kerma reflects the energy of secondary particles released by indirectly ionizing radiation at the point of interest, while the dose represents the energy absorbed by these particles. This absorption takes place at a certain distance from the origin of their production.

Figure 5 shows the attenuation of photons in their penetration through the absorber where at the surface, the kerma has a maximum value and then shows a continuous decrease, while the dose is first increasing its value and after reaching the maximum; it decreases with the same rate as the kerma (equilibrium). This behavior is due to the fact that at a certain depth, the particles from the layer above contribute to the dose where the kerma is lower because of the attenuation.

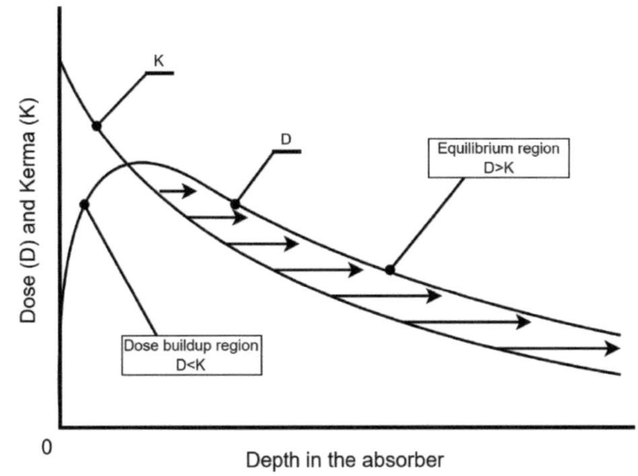

Figure 5.
The relationship between the kerma and the dose depends on the depth.

3.2 The need for assessment of biological risk

Although up to the middle of the last century, practically only the physical quantities of radiation were used for assessing the harm caused by radiation exposure to persons, it was felt that for this purpose, another set of quantities had to be introduced. Such quantities were supposed to reflect biological effects regardless of the type of radiation and irradiation geometry. This was why several weighting factors were adopted to convert pure physical quantities into quantities, which would be better related to the biological response of the exposed human body to the most common types of radiation under typical exposure conditions. The values of applicable weighting factors were derived from the investigation of some radiation accidents and incidents, and especially from extensive epidemiological studies, including those carried out on the survivors of the atomic bombing in Hiroshima and Nagasaki. Of course, these data have never been considered final since more studies led to more relevant and reliable results of the weighting factors. This was why even throughout the last few decades, there had been certain biological quantities, which serve for the radiation risk assessment used for the control of radiation exposure in order to implement the basic requirements and philosophy of radiation protection known as *justification, limitation,* and *optimization*.

As mentioned above, for the assessment of the health risk related to exposure to radiation, other types of quantities should be used. These quantities are based on specific dosimetry quantities weighted by appropriate factors in order to reflect stochastic or deterministic biological effects.

Stochastic (probabilistic) effects are random phenomena and manifest as mutations of cells and not their death. It has been found that there is no threshold dose for these effects. This concept is known as *linear no threshold model.* In most cases, any cell mutations caused by ionizing radiation will be eliminated by the body's defense; however, when this does not occur, the mutations can induce cancers (**Figure 6**).

At higher doses, the deterministic effects (tissue reactions) take place. These are known as the biological effects, which are manifested after the dose exceeds the so-called threshold level. It is not the same for all organs; the susceptibility of cells to radiation damage is described by the term radiosensitivity.

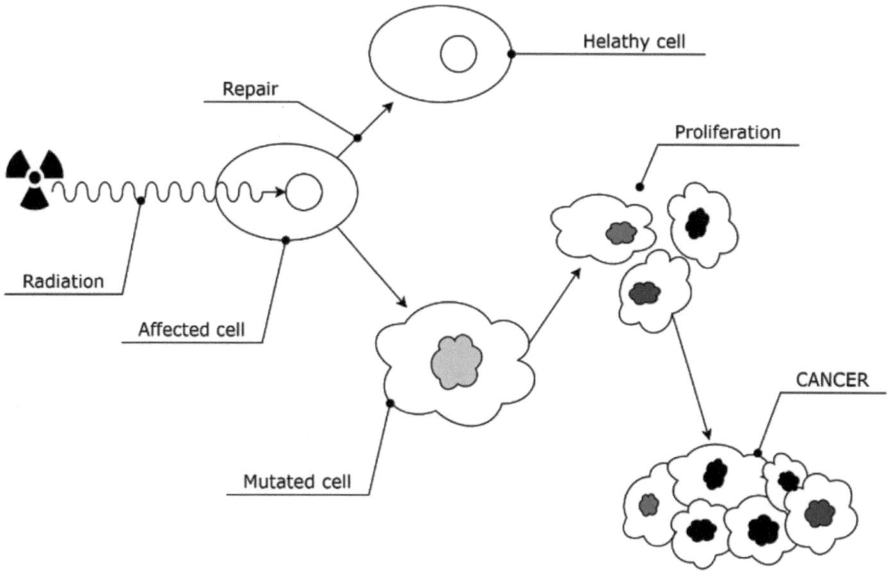

Figure 6.
Radiation-induced carcinogenesis occurs following interaction with ionizing radiation that leads to cell mutation (based on [6]).

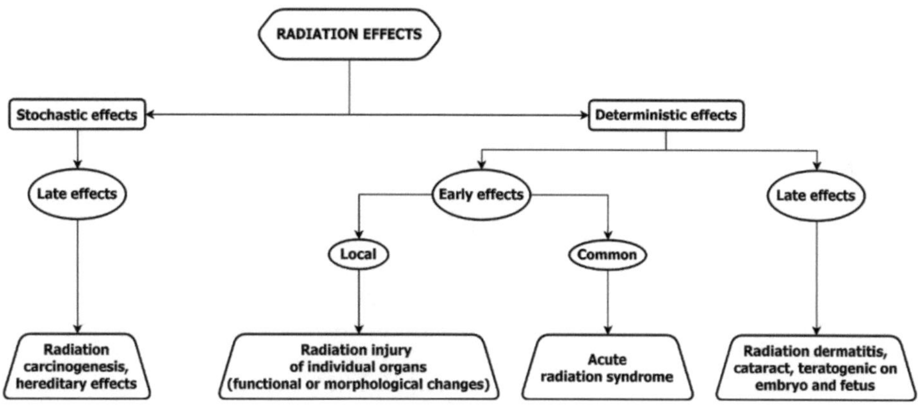

Figure 7.
An overview of biological consequences of radiation effects.

The individual categories of radiation-induced biological effects are summarized in **Figure 7**.

3.3 Quantities reflecting stochastic effects

Such quantities could be used only for relatively small doses where only probabilistic effects are expected.

The most frequently used quantities for this purpose include dose equivalent, equivalent dose, effective dose, committed effective dose, and specific operational quantities (introduced for external exposure only) approximating main radiation protection quantities.

One of the earlier quantities in radiation protection introduced for this purpose was the *dose equivalent (H)* defined at the point of interest in tissue as

$$H = D \cdot Q_F \tag{4}$$

where D is the absorbed dose, and Q_F is the mean value of the quality factor for the specific radiation at this point. The unit of the dose equivalent is sievert (Sv), which corresponds to J.kg^{-1} (multiplied by Q_F). The coefficient Q_F is one of those weighting factors mentioned above.

Since the dose equivalent is a point quantity, it itself has limited practical applications with the exception of its use in the definitions of so-called *operational quantities* (to be discussed later). More useful are the following main radiation protection quantities, namely the *equivalent dose* and the *effective dose.*

The first of these quantities *(H_T)* is defined by the summation of the average of doses ($D_{T,R}$) in a tissue or organ T caused by radiations of type R multiplied by the relevant radiation weighting factors (w_R). This quantity is quantified by the unit Sv (sievert and is defined by the expression

$$H_T = \sum_R w_R \cdot D_{T,R} \tag{5}$$

While the equivalent dose represents the health effects in individual tissues or organs, the *effective dose (E)* is a measure of radiation exposure to the whole body, which may be exposed to radiation inhomogeneously, and various sensitivities should be taken into account. This is done by so-called *tissue weighting factors (w_T)* recommended by ICRP [7, 8].

The effective dose (E) is the main quantity in radiation protection for the assessment of biological effects at low doses. It has been defined *only for stochastic effects*. The definition of the effective dose can be written in the form

$$E = \sum_T w_T \sum_R w_R \cdot D_{T,R} \tag{6}$$

here w_T is the tissue weighting factor, w_R is the radiation weighting factor and $D_{T,R}$. The unit of this quantity is sievert (Sv); more often, however, units such as mSv or μSv are used. The factor w_R is related to the Linear Energy Transfer (LET), which reflects the average amount of energy transferred per unit of distance traveled). The values of LET are usually expressed in units of keV/μm. The values of w_R for some radiations are as follows: low-LET radiation (photons, electrons, muons), 1; protons and charged pions, 2; and alpha particles, fission fragments, and heavy ions, 20. For neutrons, this factor depends on the energy [7, 8].

The LET values for some radiation are given in **Table 1**. The definition of LET is related to charged particles in any medium. As indirectly ionizing radiation, as gammas or X-rays, this quantity is associated with the secondary charged particle released by the interaction of indirectly ionizing radiation.

There is some relation between the LET and the Relative Biological Effectiveness (RBE). They both are important terms in radiation biology and reflect the relative damage that will occur under different circumstances. As LET increases, more energetic electrons are deposited closely together and thus, damage to DNA is more likely.

Since the LET is strictly speaking defined only for charged particles, its values for uncharged particles (photons and neutrons) are related to the secondary charged particles formed by this indirectly ionizing radiation.

Type of radiation	LET (keV/μm)
Co-60 gamma photons	0.3
X-ray radiation, 250 kVp	2.0
Protons, 10 MeV	4.7
Protons, 150 MeV	0.5
Recoil protons from fission neutrons	45.0
Neutrons, 14 MeV	12.0
Alpha particles, 2.5 MeV	166.0

Table 1.
The LET values of various types of radiations (based on [7]).

Type of tissues	w_T
Remainder tissues, red bone marrow, breast, colon, lung, stomach	0.12
Gonads	0.08
Bladder, esophagus, liver, thyroid	0.04
Bone surface, brain, salivary glands, skin	0.01
All tissues	1.00

Table 2.
The w_T *values of various types of radiations (based on [8]).*

The weighting factor w_T for calculating the effective dose represents a relative measure of the risk of stochastic effects that might result from exposure of a specific tissue T. It takes into account the variable radiosensitivities of organs and tissues in the body affected by radiation. The w_T values for main tissues are shown in **Table 2**.

The remainder tissues include some 13 tissues that are significantly exposed. They comprise the following tissues: adrenals, extrathoracic region, gall bladder, heart, kidneys, lymph nodes, muscle, oral mucosa, pancreas, prostate, small intestine, spleen, thymus, uterus/cervix.

Both the abovementioned quantities can be related to the unit of time as the equivalent dose rate and effective dose rate where the same units, $Sv.s^{-1}$ are used. More practical are widely used units such as $mSv.h^{-1}$ or, in the case of the effective dose, even $mSv.y^{-1}$.

Both the equivalent dose and effective dose can be used to assess stochastic effects due to the external radiation as well as internal radiation emitted by radionuclides, which entered the body and exposed its tissues and organs from inside. The overall risk attributed to the component related to the internal radioactive contamination can be assessed by the quantities *committed equivalent dose* – $H_T(\tau)$ and *committed effective dose*.

The *committed equivalent dose* represents the sum of the equivalent doses received in a particular tissue or organ of a person due to the intake of radionuclides during the period of τ, which is 50 years for adults or 70 years for children. This refers explicitly to the dose in a specific tissue or organ, in a similar way to the external equivalent dose. This quantity reflects the contribution of the internal exposure to the total equivalent dose. The committed equivalent dose $H_T(\tau)$ in a tissue or organ T is defined by

$$H_T(\tau) = \int_{t_O}^{t_0+\tau} H_T(t)dt \tag{7}$$

The *committed effective dose* – E(τ), is the sum of the products of the equivalent dose a tissue or organ, T, received from the intake of radioactive materials by inhalation and ingestion, and the appropriate tissue weighting factors, w_T, as shown in the following formula:

$$E(\tau) = \sum_T w_T H_T(\tau) \tag{8}$$

The integration time τ follows the intake at time t_0. Since the radiation weighting factor is considered to be a dimensionless factor, the unit of both the equivalent dose and committed equivalent dose is Sv (provided the dose is in Gy).

The quantity E(τ) is used rather rarely: only in the case of working with unsealed radioactive sources or an accident, which resulted in the release of substantial radioactive material contaminating the surrounding area. This may affect persons present especially by the inhalation of contaminated air.

Since the main radiation protection quantities mentioned above cannot be directly measured or monitored, specially defined quantities for assessing the risk due to external exposure have been introduced to assess this risk by means of measurable quantities. Such a set of so-called *operational quantities* have been introduced by the International Commission for Radiological Units and Measurements (ICRU) [9]. These quantities can provide an estimate or upper limit for the value of the protection quantities related to the external exposure or potential exposure of persons. They are characterized as follows:

- The *ambient dose equivalent* $H^*(d)$ represents the dose equivalent at a certain point in the radiation field that would be induced by an expanded and aligned field at a depth of d in a 30 cm standard tissue-equivalent ICRU sphere at a radius opposite to the direction of the field.

- The *directional dose equivalent* $H'(d,\Omega)$ at a given location corresponds to the dose equivalent *H* that would be induced in the extended field in the ICRU sphere at depth *d* on the radio in the defined direction of the radiation field represented by the angle *Ω*.

- The *personal dose equivalent* $H_p(d)$ was introduced for personal monitoring and is actually the dose equivalent in ICRU tissue at the relevant depth *d* below a specific point on the surface of the human body.

An overview of operational quantities is presented in **Table 3**. The basic unit of all operational quantities is Sv.

Figure 8 illustrates the position and the role of operational quantities in relation to physical quantities and radiation protection quantities. It should be noted that while operational quantities can apply only for the assessment of the exposure due to external radiation, radiation quantities represent general quantities for the quantification of the exposure resulting from both external radiation and internal exposure caused by the intake of radioactive material.

Task	Operational quantities	
	Area monitoring	**Individual monitoring**
Control of effective dose	Ambient dose equivalent, $H^*(10)$	Personal dose equivalent, $H_p(10)$
Control of doses to the skin, the hands and feet, and the lense of eye	Directional dose equivalent, $H'(0.07,\Omega)$	Personal dose equivalent, $H_p(0.07)$

Table 3.
Operational quantities proposed for dose monitoring of external exposure.

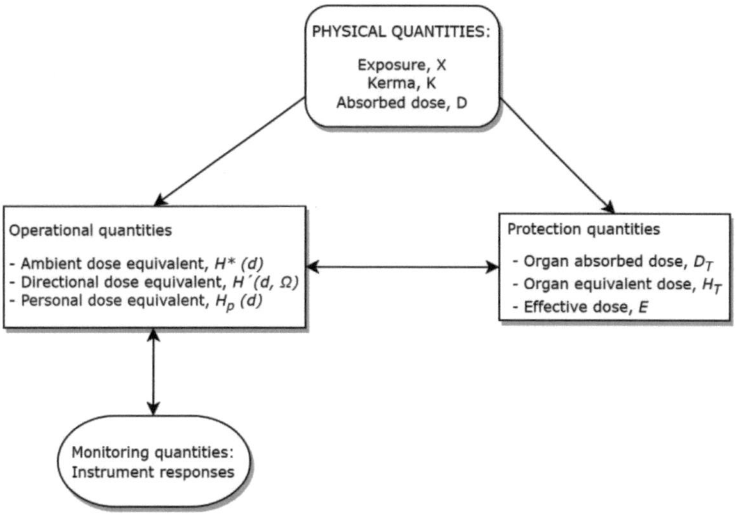

Figure 8.
Relationship between quantities used in radiation protection.

From physical quantities (exposure, kerma, dose), one can move to operational quantities using the quality factor $Q(L)$ and to protection quantities through radiation weighting factor (w_R) and tissue weighting factor (w_T). The relation between operational and protection quantities is obtained based on measurement and calculation.

3.4 Quantifies for assessment of deterministic harm

While the quantities and units for the assessment of *stochastic effects* are well elaborated and defined, this is not the case with regard to deterministic effects. Quantities aimed at the estimation of stochastic effects include both the potential harm in selected individual organs (equivalent dose) and the health impact of the irradiation of the whole body, where contributions from the exposure of individual organs are taken into account (effective dose). The stochastic effects are of primary interest at low exposure, where there are no visible signs of the reaction of tissues or organs exposed. At sufficiently higher doses where the damage caused by radiation is apparent, more interest should be paid to *deterministic effects*.

Deterministic effects (nonstochastic effects, tissue reactions) are characterized by a threshold dose that must be exceeded for effect to occur. The severity of deterministic effects increases with dose, which could result in such harms as cataracts, erythema, and sterility. The main role of radiation protection consists of keeping radiation exposure not only below the established dose limits to avoid the deterministic effects but ensure that the doses and radioactive contamination are as low as possible to achieve under the circumstances taking into account all possible specific conditions, including economic factors.

While for the assessment of stochastic effects, several quantities were defined, there has not been developed a similar approach to quantify deterministic effects [10, 11]. At present, a concept based on the RBE (Relative Biological Effectiveness) is being introduced. The relevant quantity, RBE-weighted dose (or, in short, RBE dose), is applied for this purpose [7, 12].

The RBE represents the relative absorbed dose of reference radiation (usually 250 kVp X-rays or cobalt-60 gamma rays) required to produce the same magnitude of the similar effect as the absorbed dose of the radiation in question (RBE >1 indicates that the radiation is more effective than the reference radiation). This factor is influenced by both the biological effects (cell killing, cell survival with mutations) and the LET of the radiation.

It looks like under present circumstances, the best way to call the main quantity for the assessment of the risk associated with the deterministic effects in terms of the *RBE dose* defined as

$$\text{RBE dose} = \text{RBE} \times \text{D} \tag{9}$$

with the unit Gy-Eq (gray equivalent). Therefore, a dose in Gy-Eq is the absorbed dose in Gy multiplied by a recommended RBE, which takes into account that ionizing radiation of different types and energies affects living organisms differently. The values of the RBE for some typical radiation are given in **Table 4**.

In this context, the RBE is analogous to the weighting factor w_R used to define the equivalent dose, except that in this case, the RBE is a measured quantity for a specific deterministic endpoint. In this regard, there is no equivalent to the effective dose in the case of high exposure of many tissues or organs in the body. Although the term *RBE dose* would be an appropriate choice for the quantity expressing the harm following high exposure, it is still not widely used.

There are still some inconsistencies in using units for effective dose (Sv) and RBE-dose (Gy-Eq). In some cases, the unit Sv is also wrongly used for the assessment of deterministic effects.

Type and energy of the radiation	RBE
Low-level radiations (e.g., photons, electrons)	1.0
Protons (>2 MeV)	1.5
Heavy ions (e.g., helium, carbon, neon, argon)	2.5
Neutrons <5 MeV	6.0
5 MeV	5.0
> 5 MeV	3.5

Table 4.
The RBE values for individual types of radiation (based on [8]).

3.5 Contributions from external and internal exposure

In general, radiation protection mechanisms have to provide adequate protection of persons against both external and internal exposure. The total exposure can be presented as a sum of the contribution from radiation incident on the surface of the body as well as radiation emitted by radionuclides, which enter the body through inhalation or ingestion and exposes the tissues from inside.

In order to control external radiation sources, some specific protective measures have to be in place. The radiation situation, including its impact on persons, is evaluated by appropriate quantities and other parameters characterizing the potential of the source, intensity of radiation field, and finally, the exposure of the affected person using appropriate quantities and units. The source is usually described by activity (number of radioactive decays per second) or emission (number of particles or photons emitted by the source in 1 second). The situation is illustrated in **Figure 9**.

In an analogous way, we may also characterize the circumstances in the case of personal exposure (**Figure 10**).

4. Application of radiation in medicine and some other fields

The principal objectives of radiation protection are to ensure adequate safety of persons against the harmful effects of radiation. This includes radiation workers, patients as well as members of the public. In addition, the satisfactory

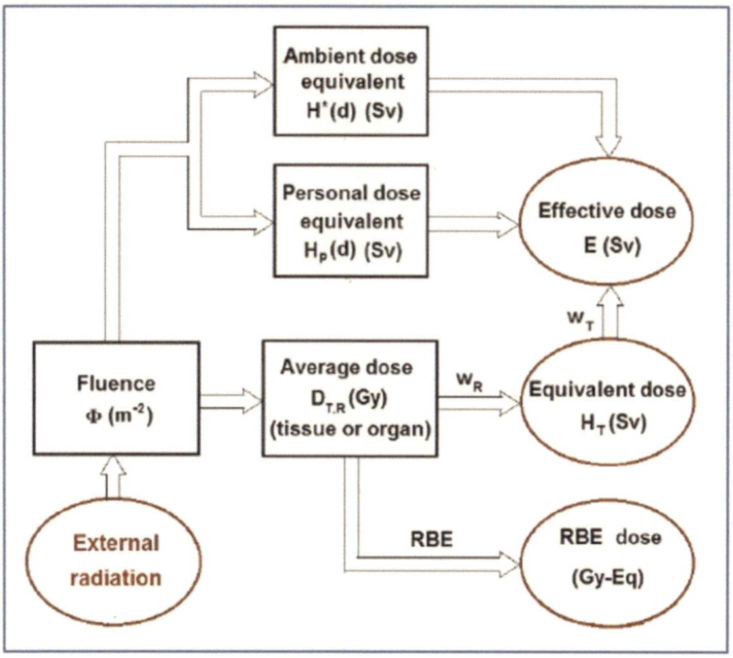

Figure 9.
Relations between various radiation protection quantities used to assess stochastic and deterministic effects following the external exposure (based on [12]).

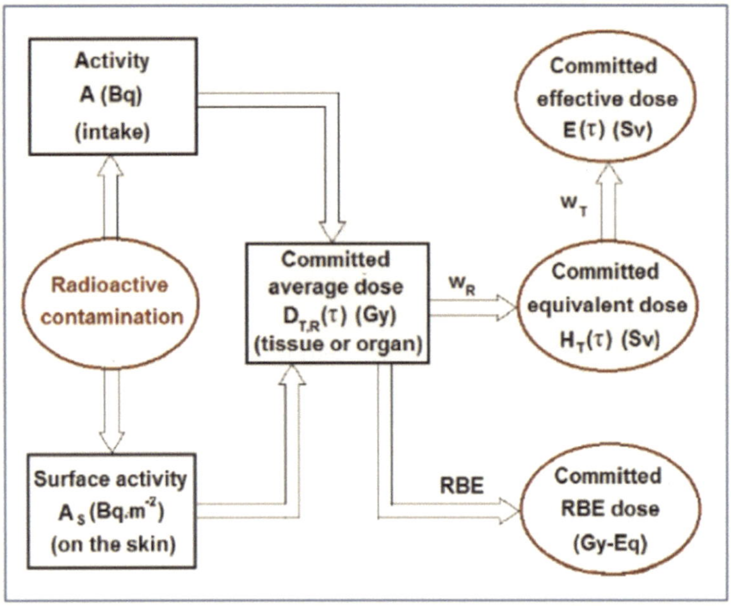

Figure 10.
Quantities characterizing personal exposure from the intake of radioactive material or from skin contamination (based on [12]).

protection of the environment, especially from its radioactive contamination, should also be taken into account. Special attention should be paid to the security of strong radioactive sources since they may be misused for terrorist and other malevolent actions.

There is no debt that exposure to radiation may cause severe hazards to workers, members of the general public, as well as to patients if the application of radiation sources is not under strict control during all their cycles, including production, transport, storage, and decommissioning. It is worth emphasizing the main role of safety and security in radiation protection. As has already been indicated above, *radiation safety* includes any operation aimed at the protection of persons against radiation emitted by the sources, while the *radiation (nuclear) security* role consists of protecting and securing radiation sources and nuclear installations against any attempt to handle or approach them by unauthorized persons including terrorists who may deliberately misuse radiation sources for malevolent actions.

Radiation and nuclear applications proved to be extremely beneficial and effective in many branches of technologies, especially in medicine, industry, and science. In a number of cases, these methods are the only feasible way to solve a problem or task. This applies to various medical fields where especially in diagnostic radiology. It would be impossible to carry out many examinations without a radiation generator or special radioactive materials (radiopharmaceuticals).

There are three main uses of radiation in medicine:

- *Diagnostic radiology* – based on photons produced by X-ray machines to obtain information from inside the patient's body. This includes conventional radiography (including fluoroscopy), computed tomography (CT), and some other modality specific to the examination purpose).

- *Nuclear medicine* – a small amount of radiopharmaceuticals is used to detect or treat disease. The type of radiopharmaceuticals is chosen or specially developed to be taken up predominantly by one organ or one type of cell in the body.

- *Radiotherapy* – utilizes high radiation doses to treat malignant and benign diseases by means of external radiation produced by X-ray tubes and specifically designed charged particle accelerators. This modality is applied to treat about half of all newly diagnosed cancer cases.

- *Sterilization* – relies on radiation, mainly gamma, X-ray, or electron, to deactivate harmful microorganisms (for example, bacteria, viruses, fungi, etc.).

Ensuring appropriate radiation protection of workers, patients, and other persons potentially affected by medical applications (e.g., members of the household of patients treated by radiopharmaceuticals) is one of the most important tasks. This is becoming more and more important at present, and it will be even more imperative in the future. The number and variety of methods used in medicine involving radiation are going continuously up. Moreover, some new diagnostic methods, especially CT modalities, are characterized by relatively high doses, which results in an increased radiation burden on the population. The situation can be illustrated by a comparison of exposure of members of the public receiving about 30–40 years ago and in some recent years (**Figure 11**). Although the data are from the USA, the situation is becoming similar in many industrialized countries, where medical exposure is responsible for more than 50% of the total annual effective dose.

Medical applications of radiation sources and radionuclides are contributing to the total exposure of the population up to 50% of the total exposure, and this is why ensuring appropriate control of dose in this field is most important. We cannot neglect, however, other areas where these technologies are used. This includes especially industrial applications where exposures are relatively low and practically always below set limits, but in the case of accidents or any other emergency, the consequences may be fatal. One has to learn lessons from such nuclear accidents as happened in Chornobyl in 1986 and Fukushima in 2011. The relevant comparison chart is shown in **Figure 12** (based on [14]).

An overview of a variety of applications of various methods and principles of radiation and nuclear technologies in the industry is presented in **Figure 13** (based on [15]).

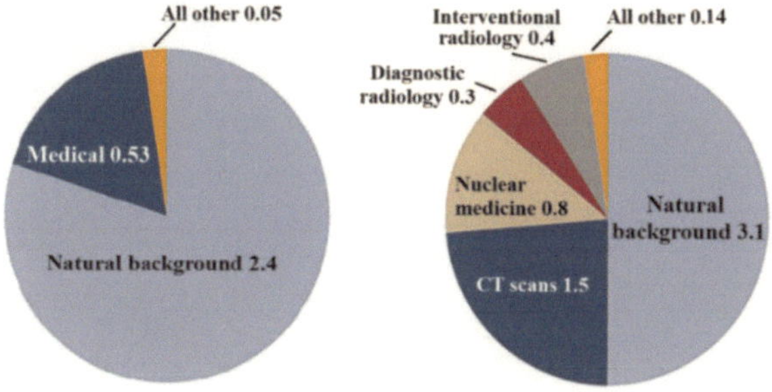

Figure 11.
Average annual effective dose/person received in 1980 (left panel) and 2006 (right panel) in the United States (based on [13]).

Chornobyl vs Fukushima

Comparison of both nuclear accidents

CHORNOBYL	FUKUSHIMA
Chornobyl disaster occurred in 1986 at the Chernobyl Nuclear Power Plant near the city of Pripyat about 130 km north of Kiev.	Fukushima accident occurred in 2011 at the Fukushima Daiichi Nuclear Power Plant in Okuma, Fukushima Prefecture
One nuclear reactor exploded in the power plant as a result of which steam ruptured.	At Fukushima Daiichi, three reactors melted down causing major reactor plant damage.
Chornobyl disaster was man-made and caused by inapropriate handling of the reactor at the low power level and the flawed reactor design	Fukushima Daiichi accident was caused by a 15-meter tsunami initiated by a massive 9.0 earthquake that hit the pacific coast of Honshu.
The disaster caused two immediate deaths and 29 more died within weeks.	No immediate deaths were recorded as a direct result of the meltdown of reactors.

Figure 12.
Difference between Chornobyl and Fukushima nuclear power plant accidents.

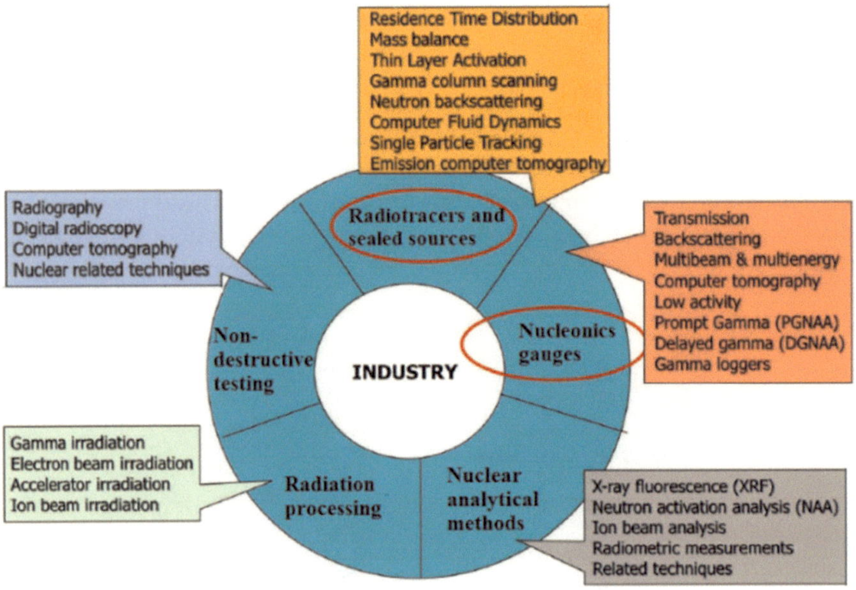

Figure 13.
Applications of radiotracer and radionuclide techniques in the industry.

5. System and legislative framework for radiation protection

The present system of radiation protection used across Europe and worldwide relies on the basic recommendations of the International Commission for Radiation Protection (ICRP). The basic conceptual framework of these fundamental materials has been constantly updated and modified, taking into account the recent development in the field.

The latest general recommendations of the ICRP were published in 2007 as *ICRP Publication 103*. At present, the ICRP is about to be reviewed and revised its last recommendations [16].

The structure and relations among the most important international committees, commissions, associations, agencies, and other related organizations are outlined in **Figure 14**. In addition to the ICRP, the most influential expert bodies among them are especially UNSCEAR (United Nations Scientific Committee on the Effects of Atomic Radiation). Other abbreviations used in **Figure 14** have the following meanings: BEIR – Biologic Effects of Ionizing Radiation, IRPA – International Radiation Protection Association, ISR – International Society of Radiology, PAHO – Pan American Health Organization, NEA – Nuclear Energy Agency, WHO – World Health Organization, FAO – Food and Agriculture Organization, BSS – Basic Safety Standards, ISO – International Organization for Standardization, IEC International Electrotechnical Commission.

The ICRP developed three main principles of radiation protection based on justification, optimization, and dose limitation.

The principle of *justification* requires that every activity related to the use of radiation sources be fully justified by a benefit that outweighs the possible risks arising from its use.

When carrying out activities leading to the exposure, it is necessary to set and maintain such a level of radiation protection that the risks arising from the use of

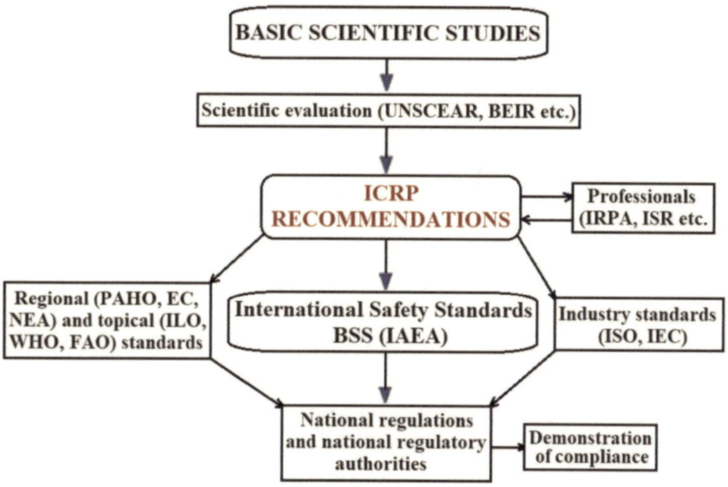

Figure 14.
The most important international expert and scientific bodies engaged in developing radiation protection recommendations and standards.

Quantity	Organ	Dose limit for exposure	
		Occupational	Public
Effective dose, E	Whole body	20 mSv/y averaged over five consecutive years, and 50 mSv in any single year	1 mSv/y
Equivalent dose, H_T	Lens of the eye	20 mSv/y, averaged over defined periods of 5 years, with no single year exceeding 50 mSv	15 mSv/y
Equivalent dose, H_T	Skin	500 mSv/y (average dose over 1 cm^2 of the most highly irradiated area of the skin)	50 mSv/y
Equivalent dose, H_T	Extremities (hands and feet)	500 mSv/y	—

Table 5.
Dose limits on occupational and public exposure (based on [17, 18]).

radiation are as low as can reasonably be achieved with regard to economic and social aspects. This is the main concept of *optimization* in radiation protection.

The *dose limitation* principle of radiation protection requires that the dose to persons should not exceed the limits introduced by the national and international standards.

Under normal or planned circumstances, the doses are not supposed to exceed the limits recommended by the ICRP (**Table 5**). The majority of countries transposed these limits for occupational and public exposure into their respective national regulations. The exposure of patients and rescue workers is controlled by specific reference doses.

6. Conclusion

Sources of ionizing radiation as well as other nuclear-related technologies have been used extensively in medicine (from cancer treatment to sterilization of medical equipment), industrial applications (nuclear power plants, production of radiopharmaceuticals, industrial radiography, radioisotope thermoelectric generators, oil well logging, industrial gauges, etc.), research, chemistry, agriculture, and in many other areas. These applications have been here for decades for the benefit of society. In their use, however, reliable safety and security measures should be introduced and followed so that any potential harm to people or the environment is kept to the minimum acceptable by the society. Here, a significant role is played by radiation protection, which should ensure the implementation of the strict regulations and safety standards aimed at the adequate protection of workers, patients as well as members of the general public against potentially harmful health effects of radiation exposure. Similar rules have been introduced to limit radioactive contamination of the environment.

Besides radiological protection of the persons in routine situations, the use of radiation sources involves several important tasks associated with the prevention and mitigation of radiological or nuclear accidents. Special attention has also to be devoted to the risk associated with possible terrorist attacks and the danger from orphan sources (lost, stolen, abandoned), which are no longer under the regulatory control.

One of the ways how to solve the present problems in radiation protection concept and philosophy could include the change regarding radiation protection quantities and units. It is believed that the limitation of the number of quantities currently in use would be undoubtedly helpful. One possible approach may rely on splitting the radiation protection quantities into two categories: the first group would include a limited number of measurable quantities that can be used in regulatory control of personal exposure, while the second category may include the continuation in using the present complicated system; this will serve for research and theoretical aspects.

Acknowledgements

The chapter has been partially supported by the project VI20192022162 carried out at the Department of Crisis Management of the PA CR in Prague.

Author details

Jozef Sabol
Department of Crisis Management, PA CR, Prague, Czech Republic

*Address all correspondence to: sabol@polac.cz

References

[1] Non-ionizing Radiation Safety. Seatle, WA, USA: Washington University; 2020. Available from: https://www.ehs.washington.edu/radiation/non-ionizing-radiation-safety [Accessed: June 2, 2022]

[2] International Ionising Radiation Trefoil Symbol. Available from: https://medium.com/fgd1-the-archive/radiation-symbol-1948-fcc2ddc33ff0 [Accessed: June 2, 2022]

[3] New ISO Standard – Ionizing Radiation Warning Supplementary Symbol. ISO; Abington, UK: Alamy, Ltd.; 2012. Available from: https://www.alamy.com/new-iso-standard-ionizing-radiation-warning-supplementary-symbol-new-image69675396.html [Accessed: June 2, 2022]

[4] Sabol J, Weng PS. Introduction to Radiation Protection Dosimetry. Singapore: World Scientific; 1995. p. 300 ISBN 981-02-2116-9

[5] Sabol J. Basic radiation protection related to the assessment of remediation measures in radioactively contaminated areas. In: Gupta DK, Voronina A, editors. Remediation Measures for Radioactively Contaminated Areas. Cham (Switzerland): Springer International Publishing AG; 2019. pp. 291-314 ISBN 978-3-319-73397-5

[6] Exam Question: Health Effects of Ionizing Radiation. Houston, USA: Radiology Physics Education; 2017. Available from: http://theimagingphysicist.com/health-effects/ [Accessed: June 2, 2022]

[7] Copeland K, Friedberg W. Ionizing Radiation and Radiation Safety in Aerospace Environments. Washington, USA: Federal Aviation Administration; March 2021. Available from: http://www.faa.gov/go/oamtechreports/ [Accessed: June 2, 2022]

[8] ICRP Publication 103. The 2007 Recommendations of the International Commission on Radiological Protection. Ann. ICRP, 2007, Vol. 37. Otawa, Canada: Ann. ICRP; 2007. 2

[9] ICRU Report 95. Operational quantities for external exposure. Journal of the ICRU. 2020;**20**(1)

[10] Sgorous G et al. MIRD commentary: Proposed name for a dosimetry unit applicable to deterministic biological effects – The Barendsen (Bd). Journal of Nuclear Medicine. 2009;**50**(3):485-487. DOI: 10.2967/jnumed.108.057398

[11] Frometa T et al. Biologically effective dose (BED) or radiation biological effect (RBEf)? In: Mughraby AM, Almayyahi B, IntechOpen, editors. Recent Techniques and Applications in Ionizing Radiation Research. London: IntechOpen; 2020. ISBN 978-1-83962-884-9

[12] Sabol J, Šesták B. Quantification of the risk-reflecting stochastic and deterministic radiation effects. In: RAD Conference Proceedings. Vol. 2. 2017. pp. 104-108. Available from: www.rad-proceedings.org [Accessed: June 2, 2022]

[13] Baselet B et al. Cardiovascular diseases related to ionizing radiation: The risk of low-dose exposure (review). International Journal of Molecular Medicine. 2016;**38**:1623-1641. DOI: 10.3892/ijmm.2016.2777

[14] Khillar S. Difference between Chornobyl and Fukushima. Marieta, GA, USA: Difference between.Net. 2021. Available from: http://www.differencebetween.net/miscellaneous/difference-

between-chernobyl-and-fukushima/ [Accessed: June 2, 2022]

[15] IAEA - RER1020 Project. To Enhance and Consolidate Regional Capability in Online Industrial Processes Using Radiotracers and Sealed Source Techniques. Warsaw: Institute of Nucl. Chem. and Technology; 2018. Available from: www.ichtj.waw.pl [Accessed: June 2, 2022]

[16] Clement C et al. Keeping the ICRP recommendations fit for purpose. Journal of Radiological Protection. 2021; **41**:1390-1409

[17] Dose limits. ICRPaedia. 2019. Available from: http://icrpaedia.org/Dose_limits [Accessed: June 2, 2022]

[18] ICRPaedia. Dose limits. ICRPaedia guide to the system of radiological protection. 2021. Available from: http://icrpaedia.org/ICRP%C3%A6dia_Guide_to_the_System_of_Radiological_Protection [Accessed: June 2, 2022]

Chapter 2

Linear Quadratic Model in the Clinical Practice via the Web-Application

Anatoly Batyan, Pavel Dziameshka, Katsiaryna Hancharova, Viktar Lemiasheuski and Aliaksandr Orgish

Abstract

The modern development and improvement of mathematical models that describe the radiobiology of processes in the body occurring under the influence of radiation every year lead to more complicated calculations related to the estimation of its impact both on the effectiveness of radiotherapy and on the possibility of making changes to the radiation treatment regimen. This significantly increases the time spent by medical physics and radiation oncologists and also requires special training of qualified specialists capable of performing such calculations. The aim of the study is to optimize calculations related to the estimation of radiation doses when the radiation treatment schedule changes, by modeling such changes with specially designed software on the basis of the theory of a linear-quadratic radiobiological model. The Web application is accessed *via* the Internet link https://hypo-calc.github.io/. As an example of using the Web application, the possible cases in clinical practice are considered.

Keywords: radiobiology, radiobiological models, linear-quadratic model, incomplete reparation, proliferation

1. Introduction

The history of the development of radiobiological models began immediately after the discovery of X-rays and is rapidly continuing at present time, overcoming an increasing number of restrictions. The practical application of biological radio models is a typical clinical practice when treating oncological diseases.

Owing to the development of radiobiological models, it has become possible to mathematically describe the biological phenomena that occur in the body under the influence of ionizing radiation. They allow for predicting the event that causes ionizing radiation in a particular cell. The practical application of radiobiological models makes it possible to calculate radiation doses and the number of fractions, compare the biological effect of irradiation under different dose fractionation regimes, and present physical quantities in the form of clinical indicators. Radiation therapy (RT) is characterized by physical and mathematical values, which are expressed by specific numerical values (dose per fraction, total radiation dose, number of RT sessions, time interval between RT sessions, etc.). But when developing and optimizing radiation treatment plans, doctors and physicists use clinical indicators (biologically effective dose, linear-quadratic equivalent dose for 2 Gy fractions, tumor control probability, normal tissue complication probability, etc.) [1, 2].

Such radiobiological models as NSD, KRE, and TDF are considered out-of-date and can be useful only for the prevention of radiation complications, but they are not effective for the destruction of malignant tumors. Also, they cannot be used to calculate the biological effect on parenchymal tissues (lungs, nervous tissue, intestines, liver, kidneys, etc.).

To date, the LQ model is the most commonly used model in clinical practice [3], but it also has limitations being a simplified model of cell damage, and it should be used with caution considering the assessment of the possible risks of complications from the dose and irradiated volume, based on the QUANTEC findings in the conditions of modern medical imaging, optimization of dosimetric planning of exposure, and new approaches to conducting RT sessions. Today, there are modifications of the LQ model [4–6], which allow calculating tolerant doses, as well as the probability of occurrence of radiation complications in tissues as a function of the volume of exposure, and single and total dose.

To achieve the main goal of radiation therapy (tumor eradication, alleviation of the patient's condition), it is necessary to deliver a dose of radiation, which is sufficient to destroy the tumor, to the volume of radiation exposure [7]. This occurs at the cost of acceptable toxicity of normal tissue, which is associated with radiation complications. The rapid development and improvement of RT planning technologies significantly affect the reduction of the negative consequences of the influence of radiation on healthy tissues and organs at risk without worsening the results of the treatment of cancers. But even with the use of the best planning technologies on modern radiotherapy equipment in accordance with high standards of treatment, for many sites, there is a high frequency of relapses and mortality from the underlying disease. A key role in this belongs to an increase in the duration of the general course of RT [8–12].

The problem of estimation of the negative impact of interruptions in radiation treatment and the ways of their compensation is regularly raised at the training courses by the International Atomic Energy Agency (IAEA) in cooperation with the Government of Russian Federation through the State Research Centre—Burnasyan Federal Medical Biophysical Centre of Federal Medical Biological Agency and the Association of Medical Physicists of Russia (AMPR). At the same time, at the present stage, it is proposed to rely on the linear-quadratic radiobiological model (LQM) theory, which has a long and complex history [13–15].

The practical application of the LQM in many institutions is an integral part of the clinical practice of cancer therapy. However, calculations related to the estimation of radiation doses when the radiation treatment schedule changes during the course of RT lead to a significant increase in the working time of medical physicists and radiation oncologists and also require special training of qualified specialists capable of conducting them.

Introducing LQM into practice for estimation of radiation doses taking into account the loss of the biological effect when modifying radiation treatment regimens, specialists face the above-mentioned difficulties. Therefore, to solve the identified issues, we have proposed the Web application that allows us to optimize the processes associated with the estimation of radiation doses when modifying the radiation treatment schedule for patients.

The aim of our study was to optimize calculations related to the estimation of radiation doses when the radiation treatment schedule changes by simulating such changes in special software created on the basis of the theory of a linear-quadratic radiobiological model.

2. Description and features of the web application

The development of the application was carried out by specialists in the field of radiobiology, medical physics, and practicing radiation oncologists on the basis of the International Sakharov Environmental Institute of Belarusian State University and N.N. Alexandrov National Cancer Centre of Belarus. The source code of the program was written by an IT developer, a specialist in applied mathematics and actuarial sciences, using JavaScript (52.2%) and HTML (47.8%) programming languages. The technical requirement for the user is to have a browser that supports JavaScript. The program is accessed *via* the Internet link https://hypo-calc.github.io/.

Web application features:

- calculation of isoeffective doses;
- calculation of the number of fractions;
- calculation of amendments for the modified treatment regimen;
- calculation of EQD_2 taking into account the interruptions in RT course;
- calculation of EQD_2 taking into account the reduction of days of treatment;
- accounting for incomplete reparation with multi-fraction irradiation per day;
- possibility of correcting errors in the release of the dose, etc.

The application is divided logically into three areas. These are the data entry area, the area of calculated values, and the treatment schedule. In the data entry area, the user sets the parameters he needs. The following cells are required to be filled in: *Dose per Fraction*, *Number of Fractions*, *Fractions proceed*, *α/β ratio*. Fields *Start of treatment*, *Recovery halftime $T_{1/2}$*, and *Use D_{prolif}* are filled in when it is necessary to take into account the duration of the course, interruptions, and incomplete reparation with multifraction irradiation per day. The *Use D_{prolif}* field becomes active when the number of days of the RT course exceeds 21 days. The appearance of the application is shown in **Figure 1**.

In the area of calculated values, the values of *Overall treatment days*, *Total dose*, *Biological Effective Dose (BED)*, and *Equivalent dose EQD_2* depend on the entered values of the *Dose per fraction* and the *Fractions*. The values in the cells *Factual gap days* and *Factual treatment days* depend on the changes made to the *Treatment Schedule*. The *Equivalent dose owing to proliferation* is calculated on condition that the cell *Use D_{prolif}* is filled.

The *Treatment schedule* is filled in automatically if the input fields are filled in correctly. Clicking on filled cells makes them empty; clicking on empty cells adds fractions. With a forced change in the number of fractions, a dose per fraction is recalculated inside the calendar cells. If the number of already treated fractions is

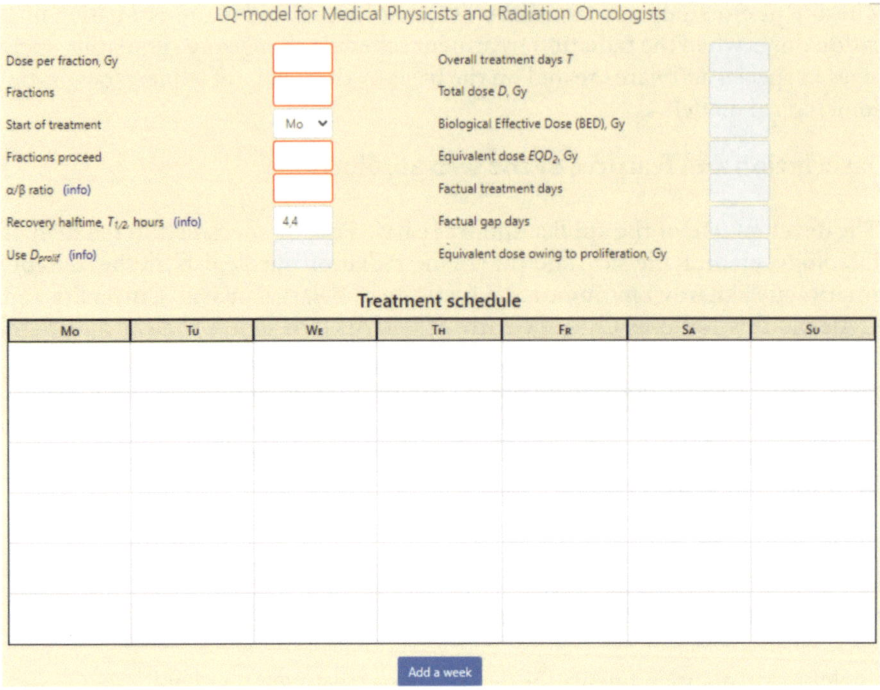

Figure 1.
Appearance of the web-application.

set, they are displayed in the *Treatment schedule* in gray. The dose in these cells is not recalculated when the number of remaining fractions changes. When pointing to a cell with the mouse cursor, it becomes available to add several factions per day by clicking on the "+" inside the cell. By clicking on Δt, the time interval between fractions can be set.

A digital copy of the application, as well as the necessary documents and materials about it, are registered and transferred for storage to the National Center for Intellectual Property of the Republic of Belarus (certificate of voluntary registration and deposit of the copyright object No. 1487-KP, act No. d20220013 dated 03/25/2022; the authors are Orgish A.N., Batyan A.N., Dziameshka P.D., Hancharova K.V., Haida A.V.).

3. Modeling clinical cases in the web application

As an example of how the application works, the following case, which is possible in clinical practice, is considered below (tasks are taken from the lectures from the training courses by the International Atomic Energy Agency (IAEA) in cooperation with the Government of Russian Federation through the State Research Centre—Burnasyan Federal Medical Biophysical Centre of Federal Medical Biological Agency "Regional Training Course on Radiobiology for Radiation Oncologists and Medical Physicists" 2018 and the Association of Medical Physicists of Russia (AMPR) "Virtual Regional Training Course on Transition from 3D Conformal Radiation Therapy to Intensity Modulated Radiation Therapy" 2021).

3.1 Calculation of isoefficient doses

It is necessary to find the value of dose per fraction for a regimen isoeffective to the classical (2 Gy per fraction in 30 fractions), implemented in 18 fractions every other day, taking into account early reactions (α/β = 10 Gy) and late complications (α/β = 3 Gy). The total treatment time does not change.

For the solution, it is necessary to fill in the active cells with data in the form as it is required in the task (**Figure 2**). Further, after filling in the *Treatment schedule*, simulate irradiation every other day. To do this, unnecessary fractions must be removed with a mouse click. The result is the value inside the calendar cells. This is 2.85 Gy for late complications of alpha beta 3 Gy. For early reactions, change the value of alpha beta to 10 and get the result of 3.06 Gy.

3.2 Calculation of the number of fractions

It is necessary to find the number of fractions during irradiation of the mammary gland at 2.67 Gy, so that this regimen is isoeffective to the classical one at 2 Gy per fraction up to 50 Gy daily, without taking into account proliferation. For the mammary gland alpha beta is 4.6 Gy; alpha beta of early skin reactions is 8.8 Gy; for late complications is 1.7 Gy.

The data of a dose per fraction, the passed fractions, and the alpha beta coefficient are entered. Next, by the selection method, the number of fractions, at which the value of the equivalent dose will be closest to 50 Grays, is substituted. In the first case, these are 17 fractions (**Figure 3**).

Then, the alpha beta for early skin reactions is changed, and the value of 18 fractions by the selection method is received (**Figure 4**).

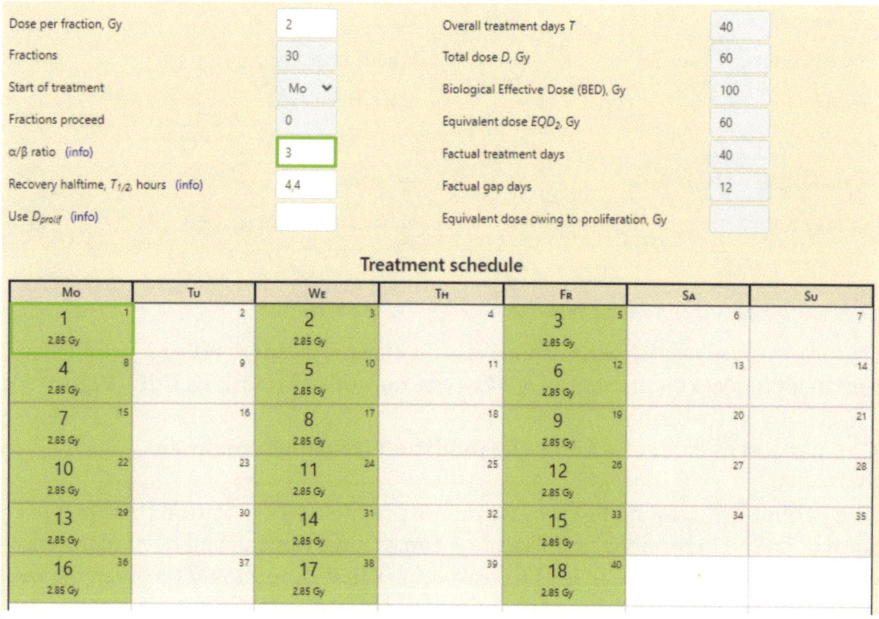

Figure 2.
Calculation of isoefficient doses.

Dose per fraction, Gy	2,67	Overall treatment days T	23
Fractions	17	Total dose D, Gy	45.39
Start of treatment	Mo	Biological Effective Dose (BED), Gy	71.736
Fractions proceed	0	Equivalent dose EQD_2, Gy	49.998
α/β ratio (info)	4,6	Factual treatment days	23
Recovery halftime, $T_{1/2}$, hours (info)	4,4	Factual gap days	
Use D_{prolif} (info)		Equivalent dose owing to proliferation, Gy	

Figure 3.
Calculation of the number of fractions. Alpha beta 4.6 Gy.

Dose per fraction, Gy	2,67	Overall treatment days T	24
Fractions	18	Total dose D, Gy	48.06
Start of treatment	Mo	Biological Effective Dose (BED), Gy	62.642
Fractions proceed	0	Equivalent dose EQD_2, Gy	51.042
α/β ratio (info)	8,8	Factual treatment days	24
Recovery halftime, $T_{1/2}$, hours (info)	4,4	Factual gap days	
Use D_{prolif} (info)		Equivalent dose owing to proliferation, Gy	

Figure 4.
Calculation of the number of fractions. Alpha beta 8.8 Gy.

Dose per fraction, Gy	2,67	Overall treatment days T	22
Fractions	16	Total dose D, Gy	42.72
Start of treatment	Mo	Biological Effective Dose (BED), Gy	109.816
Fractions proceed	0	Equivalent dose EQD_2, Gy	50.456
α/β ratio (info)	1,7	Factual treatment days	22
Recovery halftime, $T_{1/2}$, hours (info)	4,4	Factual gap days	
Use D_{prolif} (info)		Equivalent dose owing to proliferation, Gy	

Figure 5.
Calculation of the number of fractions. Alpha beta 1.7 Gy.

For an alpha beta coefficient of 1.7 Gy, the number of fractions is 16 (**Figure 5**).

3.3 Calculation of corrections for the modified treatment regimen

The patient has prescribed five sessions of preoperative radiation therapy dose per fraction of 5 Gy. On Monday and Tuesday, everything went as had been planned. On Wednesday, there was a break in the treatment. What dose should be given for the last two fractions to complete RT as planned on Friday? α/β = 10 Gr.

The data from the condition of the problem are entered. Simulate a situation in which the third fraction is skipped is simulated, and the result of 6.73 Gy per fraction is obtained (**Figure 6**).

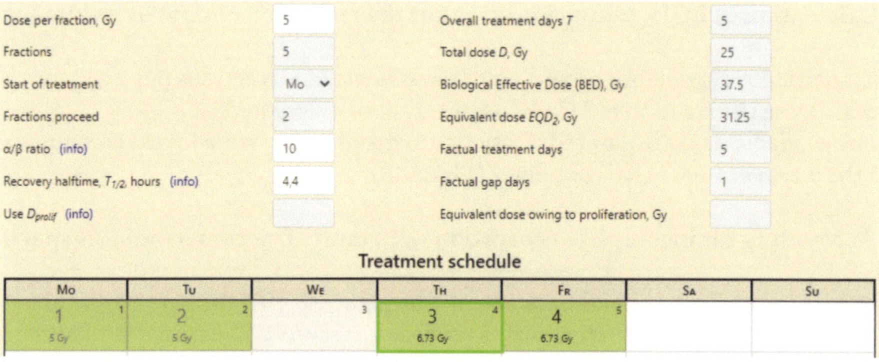

Figure 6.
Calculation of corrections for a modified treatment regimen.

3.4 Calculation of EQD_2 taking into account the interruption in RT course

Irradiation of tumors of the head and neck. The maximum dose to the spinal cord is 45 Gy. Dose on the main target is 70 Gy. Due to reactions after fraction 25, the patient was placed on a two-week break. EQD_2 is to be calculated.

The data from the condition of the problem are entered, the situation of a two-week break is simulated, and the answer of 59.5 Gy is obtained (**Figure** 7).

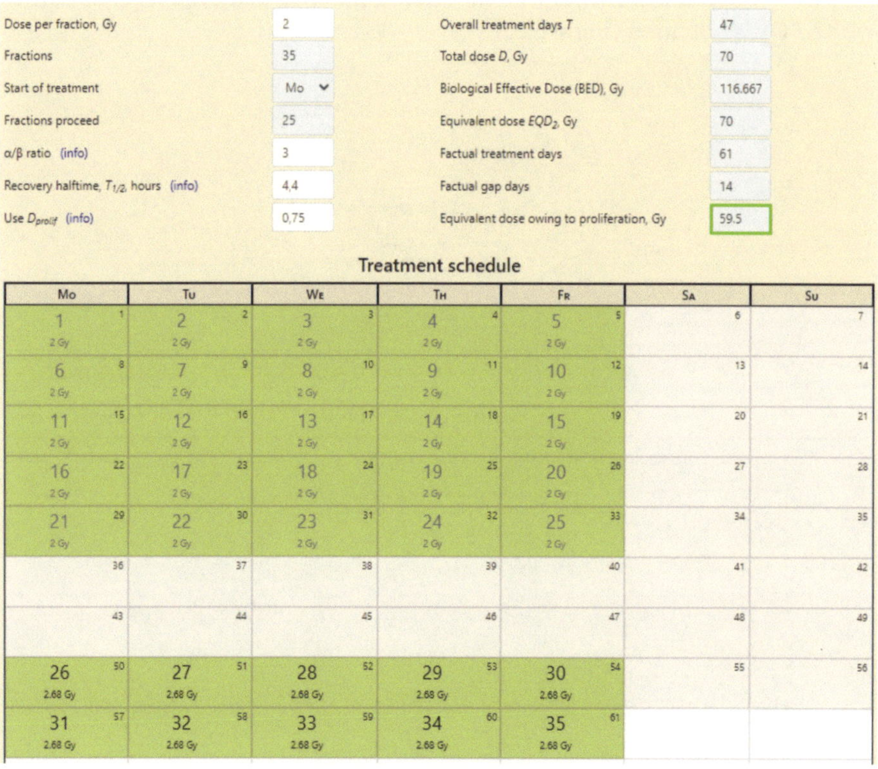

Figure 7.
Calculation of EQD_2 taking into account the interruption in RT course.

3.5 Calculation of EQD_2 taking into account the reduction of days of treatment

Irradiation is carried out according to the scheme of 6 fractions per week for 5 weeks. Dose per fraction is 2 Gr. EQD_2 needs to be calculated.

The available data are entered; factions are mandatorily transferred to Saturdays. And the answer of 64.5 Gy is obtained (**Figure 8**).

3.6 Accounting for incomplete reparation with multi-fraction irradiation per day

Irradiation of the head and neck tumor was planned with the parameters of a dose per fraction of 2 Gy 35 fractions, 5 fractions per week. The spinal cord accounts for 50 Gy (1.43 Gy per fraction). In order to reduce late complications before the treatment, it was decided to switch to 2 fractions per day with a six-hour break. It is necessary to calculate the dose per fraction and the equivalent dose to the spinal cord.

The solution to this problem consists of two stages. In the first stage, we find what dose per fraction is necessary to irradiate the tumor with an increase in the number of fractions by 2 times. To do this, we enter the data from the condition of the problem are entered. The situation, in which the number of days of treatment is doubled, is simulated. The desired value of 1.08 Gy is obtained (**Figure 9**).

At the second stage, it is necessary to pre-calculate from the proportion, which in this case is equal to the dose per fraction for the spinal cord. It is 0.77 Gy per fraction. Next, we simulate a situation in which irradiation is carried out 2 times a day. The value of a dose per fraction is changed until the values in the cells of the calendar are equal to 0.77 Gy. And the answer that the equivalent dose to the spinal cord in this case is 42.7 Gy is obtained (**Figure 10**).

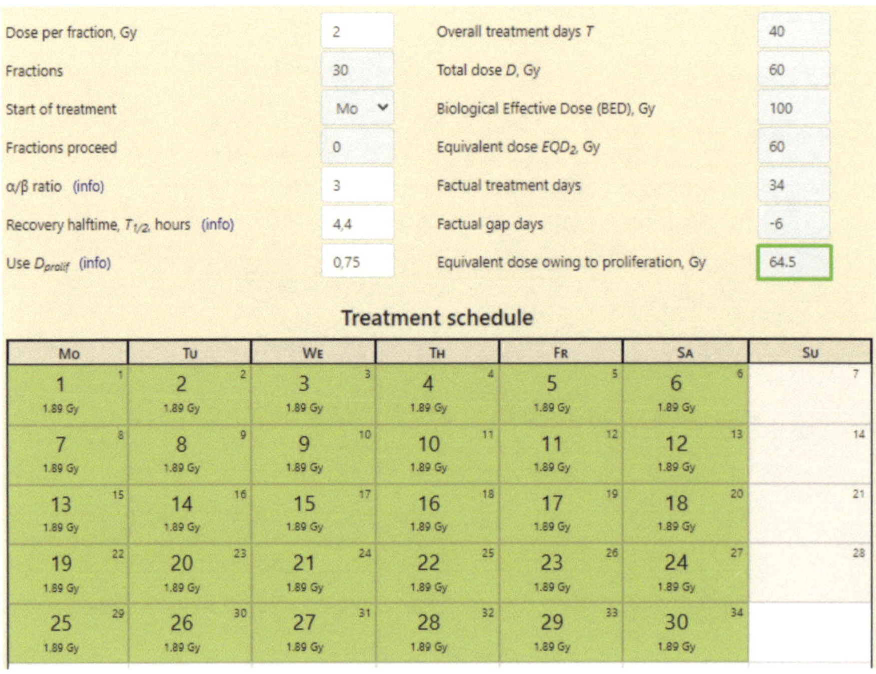

Dose per fraction, Gy
2
Fractions
30
Start of treatment
Mo
Fractions proceed
0
α/β ratio (info)
3
Recovery halftime, T1/2, hours (info)
4,4
Use Dprolif (info)
0,75
Overall treatment days T
40
Total dose D, Gy
60
Biological Effective Dose (BED), Gy
100
Equivalent dose EQD2, Gy
60
Factual treatment days
34
Factual gap days
-6
Equivalent dose owing to proliferation, Gy
64.5
Treatment schedule
Mo
Tu
We
Th
Fr
Sa
Su

Figure 8.
Calculation of EQD_2 taking into account the reduction of days of RT course.

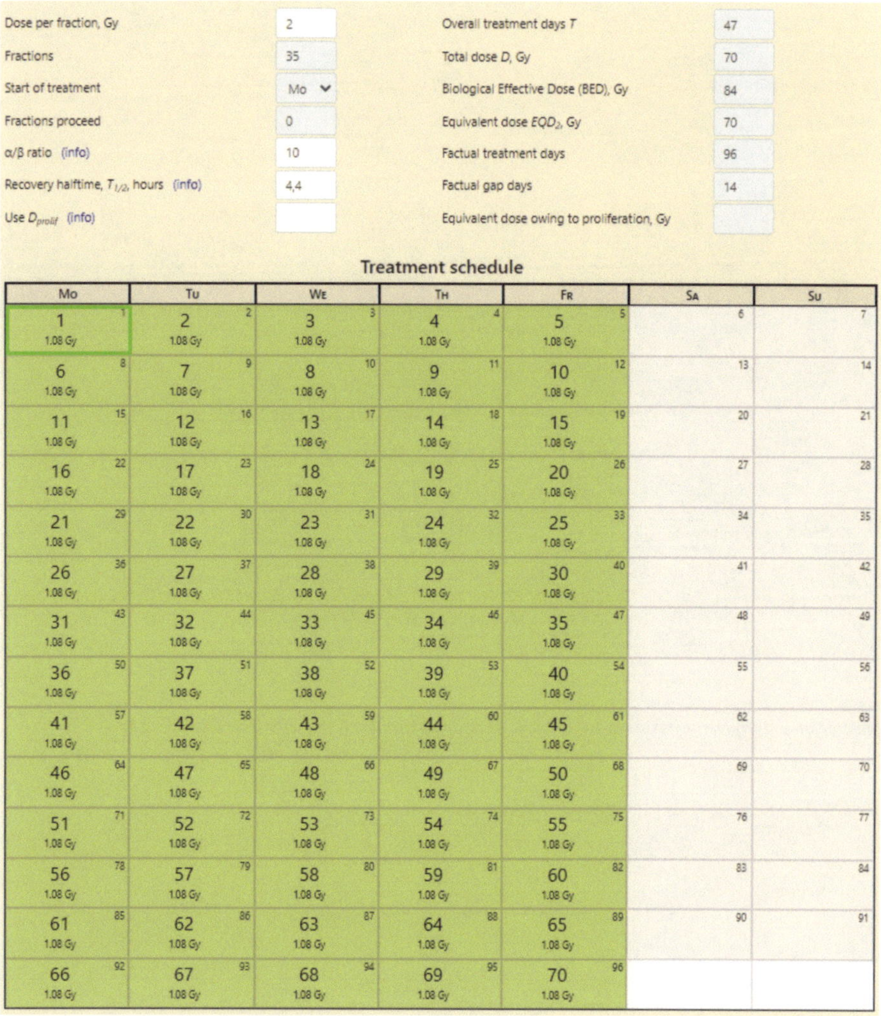

Figure 9.
Accounting for incomplete reparation with multi-fraction irradiation per day. The first stage.

3.7 Correction of errors in dose dispensing

Irradiation of a lung tumor. Dose per fraction of 2 Gy for 33 fractions is planned. After the twentieth fraction, it was found that due to an error (prescription or normalization), 1.8 Gy was supplied instead of 2 Gy. How to correct the treatment?

To find the value to which it is necessary to correct the radiation dose, it is necessary to carry out several stages of working with the application. In the first stage, the values of the already treated 20 fractions of 1.8 Gy per fraction are entered and the equivalent dose is defined (**Figure 11**).

Further, using an intermediate calculation, it is necessary to find the difference in equivalent doses between the value of the equivalent dose planned for the end of the course and the value for the first 20 fractions of 1.8 Gy: ΔEQD = 66–35.4 = 30.6 Gy. After that, the values for the remaining 13 fractions are entered into the program and the value of a dose per fraction is selected, which will correspond to the obtained value of the equivalent dose of 30.6 Gy.

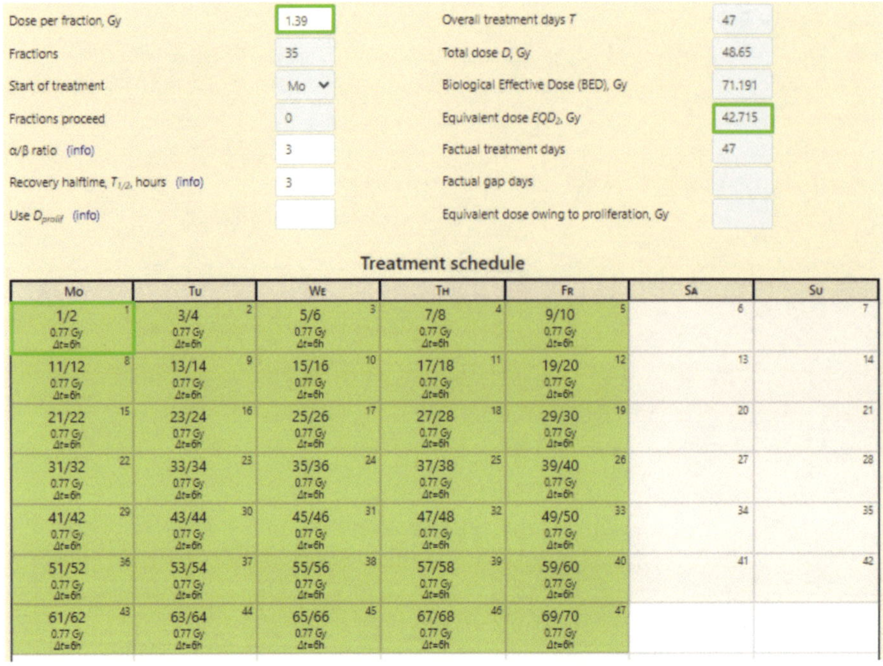

Figure 10.
Accounting for incomplete reparation with multi-fraction irradiation per day. The second stage.

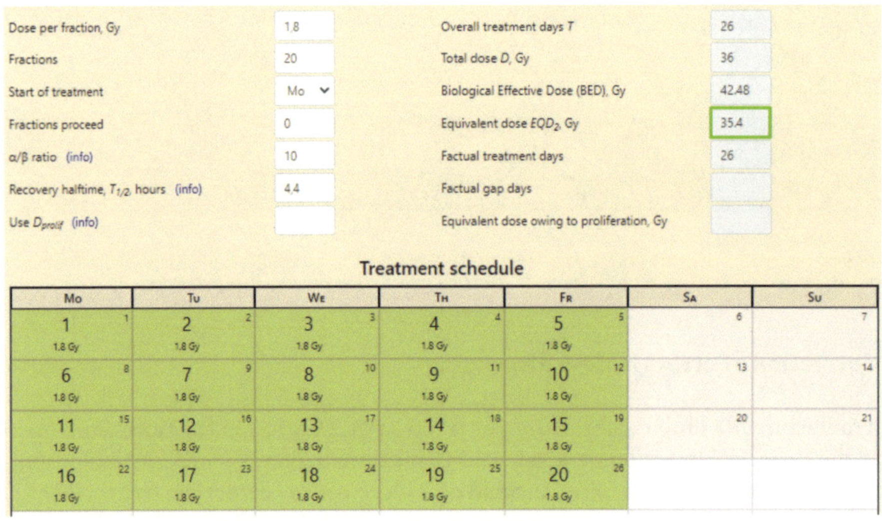

Figure 11.
Correction of errors in dose dispensing. The first stage.

The equivalent dose is to be tracked. The value of the dose per fraction is changed so that the equivalent value is 30.6 Gy (**Figure 12**). In our case, this is 2.3 Gy. This means that it is necessary to adjust the dose per fraction to a value of 2.3 Gy.

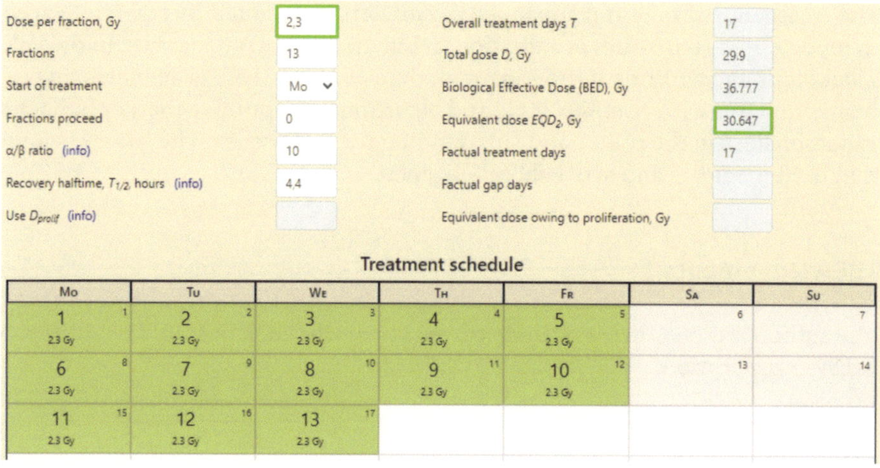

Figure 12.
Correction of errors in dose dispensing. The second stage.

4. Conclusions

Calculations related for the evaluation of the effectiveness of radiotherapy and the possibility of making changes to the radiation treatment regimen require special training of qualified specialists who are able to carry out such calculations. We have developed a computer program that allows us to optimize the work associated with the estimation of radiation doses. The application was developed with no funding. In this version, not all functions related to the evaluation of radiation doses are implemented.

The tasks in this chapter are taken from the lectures from the training courses by the IAEA in cooperation with the Government of the Russian Federation through the State Research Centre—Burnasyan Federal Medical Biophysical Centre of Federal Medical Biological Agency "Regional Training Course on Radiobiology for Radiation Oncologists and Medical Physicists" 2018 and the AMPR "Virtual Regional Training Course on Transition from 3D Conformal Radiation Therapy to Intensity Modulated Radiation Therapy" 2021. The calculation of isoeffective doses, calculation of the number of fractions, calculation of amendments for the modified treatment regimen, calculation of EQD_2 taking into account the interruptions in RT course, calculation of EQD_2 taking into account the reduction of days of treatment, accounting for incomplete reparation with multi-fraction irradiation per day, and the possibility of correcting errors in the release of the dose are considered in detail.

Description of the multicomponent and multidirectional response of the body to the action of ionizing radiation in the form of simple mathematical expressions, aimed at the treatment of malignant neoplasms within an acceptable range of complications, is a difficult task. Each modification of radiobiological models allows going deeper into biology, expanding the boundaries of applicability, and overcoming an increasing number of shortcomings. The treatment of tumor diseases is currently different for adults and children, but often there is no difference in the treatment of men and women. In addition, great importance is given to genetics, but the issues of epigenetics remain aside.

The emergence of new and advanced parameters that should be taken into account when modeling the outcomes of radiation treatment leads to an increase in the volume of calculations and additional time spent on them, so now there is an increasing need to create programs with complex logic and algorithms to optimize the assessment of the radiation dose in the tumor and surrounding normal tissues. The future belongs to personalized medicine and artificial intelligence.

Acknowledgements

The authors express their gratitude to everyone, who took part in the development of this Web application.

Conflict of interest

The authors declare no conflict of interest.

Author details

Anatoly Batyan[1], Pavel Dziameshka[2], Katsiaryna Hancharova[1*], Viktar Lemiasheuski[1] and Aliaksandr Orgish[3]

1 International Sakharov Environmental Institute of Belarusian State University, Minsk, Belarus

2 N.N. Alexandrov National Cancer Centre of Belarus, Lesnoy, Belarus

3 Sole Entrepreneur, Brest, Belarus

*Address all correspondence to: katsiaryna.hancharova@gmail.com

References

[1] Efimkina YV et al. Hypofractionated radiotherapy regimens after organ-sparing surgery for stages I–IIa breast cancer. Tumors of Female Reproductive System. 2011;**3**:45-53. (In Russ.). DOI:10.17650/1994-4098-2011-0-3-45-53

[2] Luk'yanovskii RV, Domashnikova TA, Goncharova EV, et al. Comparative analysis of radiation loads on the heart with different methods of 3D planning. Journal of the Grodno State Medical University. 2020;**18**(4):424-428

[3] Molchanova EV. Use of the LQ model and its modifications in the planning of radiation therapy for tumor diseases. A Clinical Medicine Almanac. 2008;**17**(1):354-357

[4] Klepper LY, Molchanova EV, Sotnikov VM. Calculation of the probability of a radiation complication in tissue using a modified LQED2 model as a function of radiation condition. Medical Physics. 2006;**1**(29):14-23

[5] Klepper LY, Molchanova EV. Mathematical modeling of the probability of radiation complications in therapeutic liver irradiation. Medical Radiology and Radiation Safety. 2007;**52**(2):37-42

[6] Klepper LY, Molchanova EV, Sotnikov VM. Mathematical modeling of probability of occurrence of radiation complications in lungs with their homogeneous and heterogeneous irradiation. Medical Physics. 2007;**3**(35):25-37

[7] Ministry of Health of the Republic of Belarus. Algorithms for Diagnosis and Treatment of Malignant Neoplasms: Clinical Protocol. Minsk: Professional Publications; 2019. p. 616

[8] Thames HD, Kuban D, Levy LB, et al. The role of overall treatment time in the outcome of radiotherapy of prostate cancer: An analysis of biochemical failure in 4839 men treated between 1987 and 1995. Radiotherapy and Oncology. 2010;**96**(1):6-12

[9] Dong Y, Zaorsky NG, Li T, et al. Effects of interruptions of external beam radiation therapy on outcomes in patients with prostate cancer. Journal of Medical Imaging and Radiation Oncology. 2018;**62**(1):116-121

[10] The Royal College of Radiologists. The Timely Delivery of Radical Radiotherapy: Guidelines for the Management of Unscheduled Treatment Interruptions. 4th ed. London: The Royal College of Radiologists; 2019. Ref No. BFCO(19)

[11] Yi-Jun H, Yan-Feng O-Y, Zou X, Xia L, Dong-Hua L. Chen Ming-yuan the effect of prolonged duration of intensity modulated radiotherapy for nasopharyngeal carcinoma. Frontiers in Oncology. 2021;**14**(11):648637. DOI: 10.3389/fonc.2021.648637

[12] Chang JT, See LC, Liao CT, Chen LH, Leung WM, Chen SW, et al. Early stage nasopharyngeal carcinoma: Radiotherapy dose and time factors in tumor control. Japanese Journal of Clinical Oncology. 1998;**28**(3):207-213. DOI: 10.1093/jjco/28.3.207

[13] Joiner MC, van der Kogel AJ. Basic clinical radiobiology. In: Description. Fifth ed. Boca Raton, FL: CRC Press Taylor & Francis Group; 2018. p. 350

[14] Stolbovoi AV, Zalyalov IF. Radiobiological models and clinical

radiation oncology. Oncology. Magazine named after P.A. Herzen. 2016;**6**:88-96

[15] Batyan AN, Dziameshka PD, Hancharova KV, Puhteeva IV. Evolution of radiobiological models: From concept generation to current knowledge about the effects of radiotherapy. Journal of the Belarusian State University. Ecology. 2021;**3**:49-56. DOI: 10.46646/2521-683X/2021-3-49-56

Chapter 3

Radiogenomics: A Personalized Strategy for Predicting Radiation-Induced Dermatitis

Beatriz Regina Lima de Aguiar, Eliete Neves Silva Guerra and Paula Elaine Diniz dos Reis

Abstract

Although radiation therapy (RT) planning and execution techniques have evolved to minimize radiotoxicity to a considerable extent, adjacent tissues still receive a substantial dose of ionizing radiation, resulting in radiotoxicities that may limit patients' quality of life. Depending on the location of tissue injury and the severity of the cellular response, there may also be a need to interrupt RT, thus interfering with the prognosis of the disease. There is a hypothesis that genetic factors may be associated with individual radiosensitivity. Recent studies have shown that genetic susceptibility accounts for approximately 80% of the differences in toxicity. The evolution of genomic sequencing techniques has enabled the study of radiogenomics, which is emerging as a fertile field to evaluate the role of genetic biomarkers. Radiogenomics focuses on the analysis of genetic variations and radiation responses, including tumor responses to RT and susceptibility to toxicity in adjacent tissues. Several studies involving polymorphisms have been conducted to assess the ability to predict RT-related acute and chronic skin toxicities, particularly in patients with breast and head and neck cancers. The purpose of this chapter is to discuss how radiogenomics can help in the management of radiotoxicities, particularly radiodermatitis.

Keywords: neoplasms, radiation therapy, radiodermatitis, radiation genomics, single-nucleotide polymorphism

1. Introduction

1.1 Radiation therapy (RT)

Radiation therapy (RT), a local therapeutic modality for cancer, uses beams of ionizing radiation to inhibit or control the growth of tumor cells and can be practiced alone or in conjunction with other therapies [1]. It is used in approximately 50–60% of cancer treatments for curative and palliative purposes [1–3].

There are two modalities of RT, namely brachytherapy and teletherapy. Brachytherapy uses a source of ionizing radiation that is in contact with tumor tissue and allows higher doses of radiation to reach the target tissue [4, 5]. Teletherapy, also called external RT, is the most common type of RT and is performed using machines, typically linear accelerators, which allow a source of ionizing radiation to be positioned at a certain distance from the patient and programmed to focus on the tumor [4, 5].

1.1.1 Mechanism of action of RT

For a normal cell to be able to multiply, the cell cycle takes approximately 10–20 hours [6]. Tumor cells tend to proliferate faster. During the G2 and mitotic (M) phases of the cell cycle, chromatin is more compact and hinders the action of repair enzymes, thereby increasing the probability of DNA damage [3]. Therefore, these are the two phases of the cell cycle (G2 and M) in which cells are the most radiosensitive [3, 4, 6, 7].

In addition to DNA damage, other mechanisms of cell damage can result from the use of ionizing radiation, which induces cell death. The type of cell death induced by ionizing radiation depends on the cell type, cell cycle stage, DNA damage repair capacity, ionizing radiation dose, and cellular microenvironment [3, 7, 8]. This can occur through direct or indirect mechanisms.

The direct mechanism of cell death induced by RT involves the absorption of energy by the cellular biological environment, and this energy interacts directly with DNA and proteins, causing damage that can occur up to a time after tissue irradiation [4, 6, 8]. In the indirect mechanism, ionizing radiation interacts with molecules that constitute the cell environment, primarily water, increasing the concentration of free radicals that can enhance radiosensitivity and promoting cellular damage [4, 6]. Double-strand DNA breaks can also be induced by reactive oxygen species, which are naturally produced during cellular metabolism [7].

The recognition of DNA damage induced by ionizing radiation promotes the activation of a cascade of signals that, depending on their function, will determine whether the fate of cell repair, cell cycle progression, or apoptosis [9]. Furthermore, increasing the concentration of reactive oxygen species can activate genes that induce tissue inflammation or increase oxidative stress, thereby affecting radiosensitivity [9]. The inflammatory cascade can also be induced by exposure to ionizing radiation [1].

Cellular response to radiation is also regulated by gene activation cascades and signal transduction proteins, which involve the *PI3K/AKT, MAPK/ERK, NF-κB* and *TGFβ* pathways [10]. The *MRE11-RAD50-NBS1* complex and *53BP1*, *γH2AX*, and *MDC1* genes repair DNA end fragments [9]. The *ATR* and *ATM* genes are responsible for activating DNA repair processes by homologous recombination and non-homologous end splicing, respectively, after double-strand breakage [8, 9, 11]. These genes also interact with other genes that are essential checkpoints for verifying the integrity of genetic material in the phases of the cell cycle [9, 11]. If DNA damage is significant, cell death occurs [8]. Any alteration in the function of the genes that participate in the pathways, which regulate cellular responses to radiation, influences DNA repair, cell cycle progression, and cell death by apoptosis.

Considering that tumor cells multiply faster than normal tissue cells, they tend to go through the G2 and M phases of the cell cycle more often. For RT to be effective in controlling the growth and multiplication of tumor cells, the planned total ionizing radiation dose is subdivided into daily doses (dose fractionation). RT fractionation regimens aim to reach the largest number of tumor cells in the most radiosensitive phases of the cell cycle (G2 and M), thereby increasing the therapeutic effect of ionizing radiation. The dose of ionizing radiation absorbed per unit mass in RT is defined as Gray (Gy) [5]. From the first dose of ionizing radiation, free radicals, reactive oxygen species, double-strand DNA breakage, and recruitment of the inflammation cascade are generated [1]. Total dose fractionation also aims to minimize adverse effects on healthy tissues adjacent to the tumor [5].

1.1.2 Adverse effects of RT

Toxicity resulting from exposure to ionizing radiation is very common [1, 2]. Considering that some healthy tissues, including the skin and mucous membranes, have a high proliferation capacity, fractioned doses also reach these tissues, promoting adverse reactions [1].

Adverse effects of RT are characterized by reactions that occur in tissues adjacent to the tumor or in contact with ionizing radiation during dose administration. These adverse effects can be acute or chronic, depending on the time of onset [7].

Acute adverse effects appear during RT or up to 3 months after completion in tissues with a high proliferation capacity [3, 4, 7]. For example, tissues such as the skin and mucous membranes are frequently affected [3, 4, 7]. The chronic effects appear from 3 months after the end of RT to years later, affecting tissues composed of cells with lower proliferation capacity such as cardiac, muscular, and subcutaneous tissue [3, 4, 7, 12].

Depending on the severity of the acute reactions, treatment may need to be interrupted [7]. These reactions cause pain and discomfort and may negatively impact patients' quality of life [3].

1.2 Acute radiation dermatitis (ARD)

Acute radiation dermatitis (ARD) is a skin reaction with a high incidence that affects cancer patients undergoing RT for up to 3 months after the end of the treatment [13, 14]. Approximately 95–100% of cancer patients have some degree of ARD during RT, which is very common in patients treated for breast and head and neck cancer [15–17]. The first effects of ionizing radiation on the skin are expected to appear 2–4 weeks after the first dose of RT [15].

ARD usually starts with hyperpigmentation of the irradiated area, followed by mild or transient erythema, intense erythema, dry desquamation, and moist desquamation, and in more severe cases, leads to hemorrhage, necrosis, and ulceration (**Figure 1**) [15]. Generally, RT is interrupted when patients present with disseminated moist desquamation and the skin tissue does not progress to more severe reactions.

1.2.1 Pathophysiology

The pathophysiological mechanism underlying ARD development is similar to that of the mechanism of ionizing radiation on the tumor, i.e. through direct and indirect DNA damage mechanisms. The effects of RT on skin tissue are cumulative and add up to each fraction of the ionizing radiation received [15, 18].

Tissue injury occurs through alterations in the double-stranded DNA of epithelial cells or through an increase in the concentration of reactive oxygen species in the intracellular environment [15, 16]. These lesions primarily affect the basal cells of the epidermis, which cannot self-renew in sufficient time to reconstitute the tissue [15]. Furthermore, ionizing radiation promotes the activation of the inflammatory cascade in the skin tissue [15, 16, 18].

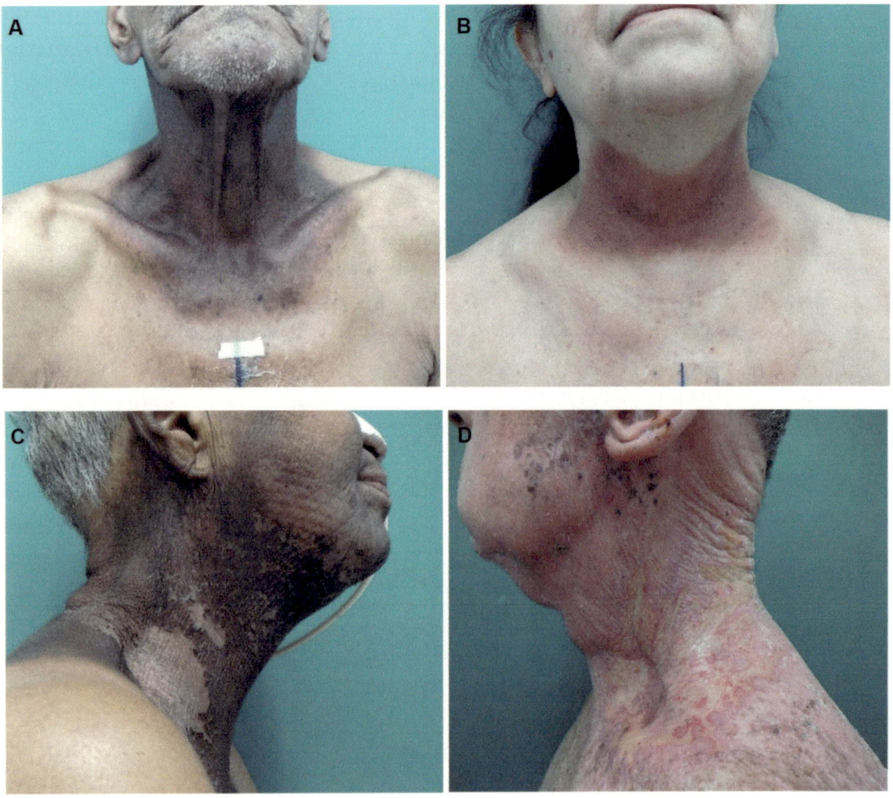

Figure 1.
Signs of ARD in head and neck cancer patients: A) hyperpigmentation; B) erythema; C) dry desquamation; D) moist desquamation. Source: Digital collection of the interdisciplinary Laboratory for Applied Research to clinical practice in oncology (LIONCO).

Skin hyperpigmentation occurs due to excessive stimulation of melanin production triggered by exposure to ionizing radiation [14, 15].

Local erythema starts soon after the first fraction dose of RT and is more intense around the second week due to vasodilation and increased vascular permeability [13–15]. This then initiates an inflammatory reaction with the release of chemokines and cytokines (primarily interleukins and TNF-α), which control endothelial cell adhesion and recruit immune cells [15]. This process can be observed as the manifestation of intense erythema [15].

Dry desquamation usually appears at an accumulated dose of approximately 30 Gy [14], between the third and fourth week [13]. This occurs as a result of a rapid compensatory attempt to renew epidermal basal cells, which occurs faster than the elimination of damaged epidermal cells [15]. In addition, RT promotes lesions in the cells of the sebaceous glands and hair follicles, which causes increased dryness of the skin and loss of hair in the treated area [15]. When the entire basal layer is destroyed, moist desquamation occurs after approximately 4–5 weeks of treatment [13] with barrier disruption and exudate production [15].

It is important to emphasize that these cellular reactions will be observed in the skin corresponding to the irradiated area and do not necessarily need to occur gradually. In addition, the time to the onset of each degree of reaction may vary among patients. Scales are generally used to measure and monitor the evolution of

ARD during treatment. The Common Toxicity Criteria for Adverse Events (CTCAE) scale [19] and the Radiation Therapy Oncology Group (RTOG) scale [20] are widely used.

1.2.2 Clinical management

Several regular skin care guidelines, including cleaning the irradiated area daily using neutral soap and warm water without friction on the skin, drying gently, keeping the treatment area protected from sun exposure, and wearing looser clothes to avoid friction [13, 14, 16], are well documented in literature and patients should be oriented to these before beginning RT.

Although there are several skin care recommendations for the treated area before and during RT, these measures do not definitively prevent the development of ARD. However, it is still no consensus in the literature on the products that are effective in preventing ARD [7, 21, 22]. Therefore, the use of predictive mechanisms for the development of ARD would be a useful tool for improving treatment planning.

1.2.3 Risk factors and individual Radiosensitivity

The following risk factors predispose patients undergoing RT to develop severe ARD:

- Treatment-related factors, including volume of treated area, tumor location (superficial or deep), total dose of ionizing radiation, fractional dose, duration of treatment, use of boost, and combination with other cancer treatment modalities [13, 15, 23].

- Patient-related factors, including exposure to solar radiation (UVA and UVB), skinfolds, humidity in the irradiated region, smoking, alcohol consumption, nutritional status, body mass index (BMI), sensitivity of the exposed skin, preexisting skin diseases, and genetic factors [13, 15, 23].

Risk factors for ARD can be considered determining factors for individual radiosensitivity. Radiosensitivity refers to the susceptibility to adverse effects resulting from exposure to ionizing radiation.

One of the challenges associated with planning the treatment of cancer patients is the identification of factors that influence the increase in individual radiosensitivity and decrease in tissue repair capacity [2, 3, 24]. However, patients with similar risk factors and treatment regimens may have different degrees of ARD. Furthermore, literature suggests that genetic factors can influence the tissue response to ionizing radiation [2].

1.3 Genetic markers and radiotoxicity

Research on factors that influence the development of adverse reactions to RT has investigated the contribution of genetic factors to these reactions [25]. This concept emerged from the identification of syndromes that make individuals more sensitive to ionizing radiation, such as the ataxia-telangiectasia syndrome resulting from mutations in genes that respond to DNA damage and repair [26, 27]. Thus, biomarkers may help in treatment planning.

Thus, radiogenomics has emerged as an area of study that aims to identify biomarkers that can predict adverse reactions in cancer patients undergoing RT or to identify individuals who are more susceptible to developing a severe degree of these reactions [3, 10, 28].

Biomarkers are molecules/biomolecules that can be measured in biopsy samples, body fluids, and feces to indicate the state of normal metabolic processes, diseases, and responses to a particular treatment [3, 29].

In 2009, the Radiogenomics Consortium (Manchester, United Kingdom) was established and supported by the National Cancer Institute (NCI) [30]. In 2019, 133 institutions from 33 countries participated in the Consortium [31]. The objective of the Radiogenomics Consortium was to establish collaborations between countries so that studies on the association between biomarkers and adverse reactions to RT could be carried out in large cohorts [10, 32] in order to identify molecular pathways that participate in the development of adverse reactions to RT and variants in the genome that are capable of predicting the development and severity of these reactions [10, 30, 31, 33].

The primary biomarkers studied by the Radiogenomics Consortium are single-nucleotide polymorphisms (SNPs) [31, 34]. SNPs are considered suitable genetic markers in studies on their association with phenotypic characteristics, as they are frequent in populations and are easily genotyped [35]. Furthermore, samples for single-nucleotide polymorphism (SNP) screening can be obtained from any normal tissue, considering that polymorphisms are present in all normal cells, including blood cells [33].

1.3.1 Single-nucleotide polymorphism

The DNA sequences of any two individuals in the world are approximately 99.9% similar to each other [36, 37]. Variations in only 0.1% of the genome make individuals phenotypically different from each other [3, 37–39]. Among these 0.1% variations, approximately 99% are due to SNPs [40].

Mutations and SNPs are genetic variants present at specific positions in the DNA sequence. SNPs are considerably common among individuals and have a probability of 1% or more of being identified in an individual, whereas "gene mutation" refers to variations in the DNA that are present in less than 1% of the population [36, 37]. Although these definitions are well established, the nomenclature remains confusing [36]. Condit et al. [41] suggest the use of the terms "genetic variant" or "genetic alteration" to replace the definitions of mutations and polymorphisms that can be complemented with the terms "pathogenic" or "benign" [36, 42]. However, the establishment of a generalist nomenclature has still been discussed.

SNPs are genetic variants that occur with the replacement of a single nucleotide in a genome sequence [27]. The variation that results in SNP can occur in non-coding regions such as intergenic and intron regions, which will not promote phenotypic changes, and in the exon coding region, which may or may not modify the gene function and consequently the phenotype (**Figure 2**) [35, 37, 44]. Although exchange of a nucleotide at a specific position can be performed by any other nucleotide (C, G, A, or T), SNPs are generally biallelic [35, 45].

To understand mechanism by which SNPs occur in DNA and their impact on the phenotype, let us look at the following example:

On chromosome 19, the locus that encodes *TGFβ* is most commonly found in exon 1, at a guanine nucleotide (G) at position 869. On the complementary strand of DNA, G pairs with a cytosine (C) encoding the amino acid Proline (Pro) at codon 10

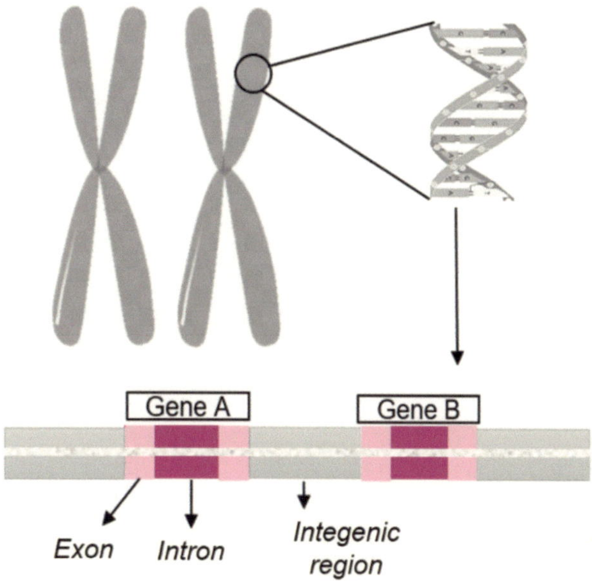

Figure 2.
Schematic representation of the non-coding (intron) and coding (exon) region of a gene. Generated with reference to the schematic representation by Alberts et al. [43].

(**Figure 3A**). Considering that it is most frequently found in the population, C, in this example, is called the wild allele. However, in some individuals, an exchange of G for adenine (A) at this position has been observed (**Figure 3B**). This exchange also leads to a change in the complementary strand of DNA, that is, the exchange of C for thymine (T), thus encoding the amino acid leucine (Leu) (**Figure 3C**). In this example, the T allele is called a variant allele because it is less frequent in the population. Considering that this allelic variation (G > A) is present in more than 1% of the population, it is called an SNP. This *TGFβ* SNP is referred to as Pro10Leu or encoded as rs1800470.

The human genome is diploid; that is, we inherited 23 chromosomes from the father and 23 from the mother, which are organized into pairs by similarity to each other. This organization into pairs of similar chromosomes is called homologous chromosomes, which have very similar nucleotide sequences. Therefore, SNPs can occur on one chromosome or on a homologous pair of chromosomes, and hence, they can be classified as homozygous for the wild allele, homozygous for the variant allele, or heterozygous (**Figure 4**).

1.3.2 Techniques for studying single-nucleotide polymorphisms

The candidate gene approach has been used to assess the association between SNPs and adverse reactions to RT. For this, genes that are already known to participate in the molecular mechanism underlying the development of adverse reactions are selected [39, 46]. Seibold et al. [47] performed a study of candidate genes involved in oxidative stress to verify their ability to predict late toxicity in 753 breast cancer patients who underwent RT. The study showed that breast cancer patients carrying the rare allele for the SNP rs2682585 in *XRCC1* had a low occurrence of late cutaneous toxicities (OR: 0.77; 95% CI: 0.61–0.96; p = 0, 02) [47]. The association of this SNP with late skin toxicity in breast cancer patients undergoing RT has been validated by

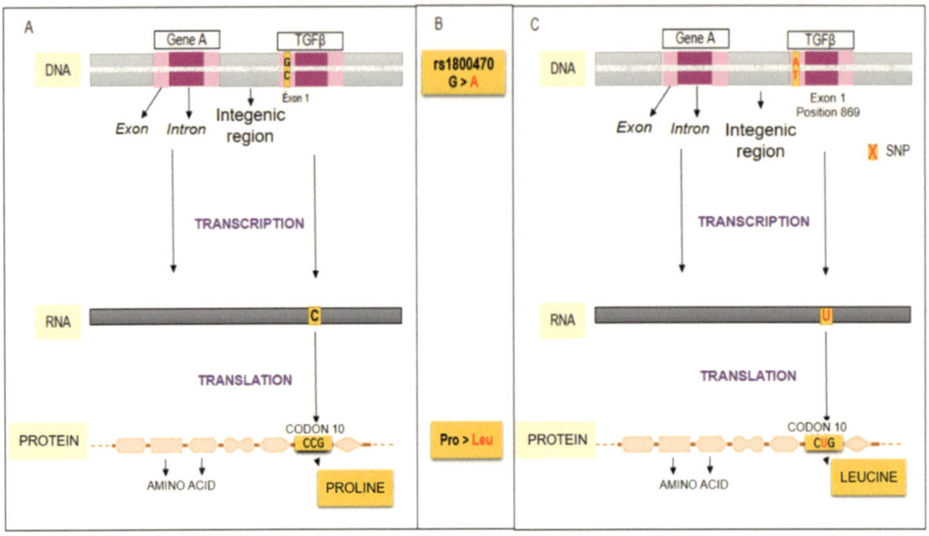

Figure 3.
Schematic representation of the rs1800470 SNP in TGFβ. A) the nucleotide sequence that makes up TGFβ will be transcribed into RNA and one of the strands will be translated into a protein that has proline (pro) at codon 10; B) rs code of the SNP in TGFβ (rs1800470) and the respective exchange of base (G > a) and protein (pro>Leu); C) SNP occurs at position 869, of exons 1, of TGFβ (G > a) and originates a complementary strand with a thymine at this position. Thymine will be transcription into uracil which will give rise by translation to a protein with leucine (Leu) at codon 10.

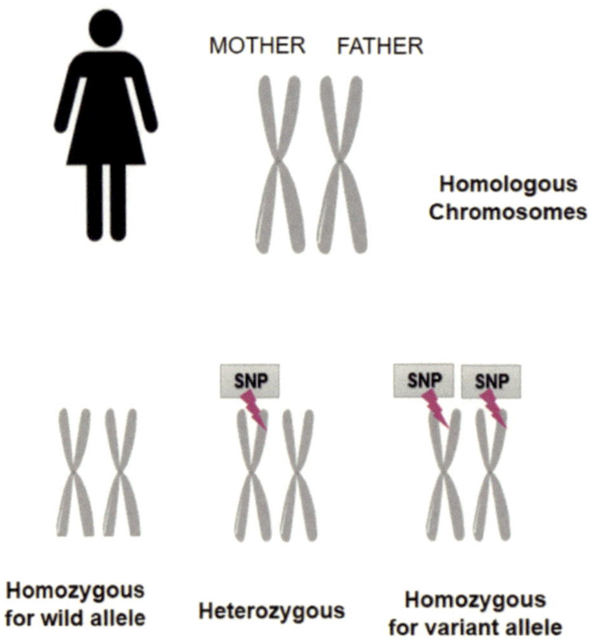

Figure 4.
Classification according to the occurrence of SNP in homologous chromosomes.

members of the Radiogenomics Consortium [28]. An important challenge in developing such research is that researchers must have basic knowledge about molecular biology and the effects of ionizing radiation on DNA [27].

Other techniques that investigate susceptibility genes, including genome-wide linkage studies (GWLS) and genome-wide association studies (GWAS), are used to conduct a broader investigation of all genes rather than an investigation of those genes already known to participate in molecular pathways involved in disease development [37]. These techniques are based on full-genome scanning and are extremely useful for investigating polymorphisms that may be associated with adverse reactions to RT [39, 46]. However, they are rarely used in studies on the association between polymorphisms and ARD. The Radiogenomics Consortium aims to obtain resources to enable the evaluations in large cohorts using the GWAS technique [30, 32].

2. The association of SNPs with acute radiation dermatitis prediction

Studies have investigated the association between SNPs and the severity of ARD that developed at the end of RT, primarily in patients receiving RT for head and neck and breast cancer.

2.1 Breast CANCER patients

A systematic review [48] of 16 cohort studies at low risk of bias, with a total of 4742 breast cancer patients treated with radiotherapy, summarized the data on whether SNPs predict ARD. Before the start of radiotherapy, all studies collected blood samples to identify SNPs and considered any manifestation of moist desquamation as a severe degree of ARD. Several studies included in this review presented statistically significant associations between SNPs and ARD. Twenty-nine SNPs were significantly associated with increased susceptibility to developing severe ARD and fifteen SNPs were significantly associated with decreased susceptibility to severe ARD ($p < 0,05$) However, it was not possible to compare the results in different samples because these associations were found in only one individual study. Furthermore, a wide variety of SNPs are being evaluated in individual studies, which makes it difficult to synthesize the data in a meta-analysis.

Considering the individual studies included in this systematic review, two SNPs had a significant association in more than one study, but with controversial results.

The rs8193 SNP in *CD44*, with CT and CT + TT genotypes, was associated with a 2.68-fold and 2.31-fold increase, respectively, in the risk of developing severe ARD in one study [49]. However, another study [50] found that the recessive model (TT) individually decreased the risk of developing severe ARD by 52%. *CD44* is a gene that involves transmembrane cell adhesion that is highly expressed on the surface of the dermis; however, its mechanism of action in healing remains unclear [51–56]. The meta-analysis found that the CC genotype is associated with the development of mild ARD, which did not manifest moist desquamation, and the CT genotype is associated with the development of severe ARD. However, with considerably low evidence certainty, further studies are required to investigate this SNP.

The rs3744355 SNP in *LIG3* was associated with the occurrence of ARD in one study ($p = 0.0046$) [57], but the authors did not report further information. Another study [50] found that the dominant pattern of this SNP was associated with a 68% decrease in the risk of developing severe ARD. *LIG3* acts on the DNA repair pathway by base excision, resulting from exposure to reactive oxygen species produced by exposure to RT [12, 57, 58].

Despite being evaluated in eight studies that composed this systematic review, the SNP *XRCC1* (rs25487) demonstrated a prevalence of 31% in breast cancer patients;

however, the data were not sufficient to allow the assessment of the association of this SNP with the severity of ARD.

The most prevalent SNPs were rs1800469 in *TGFβ1* (41%) and rs3957356 in *GSTA1* (36%). *TGFβ1* encodes a protein that acts on the inflammatory response pathways by repairing DNA lesions; however, it is not yet known whether SNPs can affect the function of this protein [59, 60]. *GSTA1* is involved in the production of reactive oxygen species, and SNPs can promote increased radiosensitivity through indirect damage to the DNA of skin cells [61]. Meta-analysis of genome association studies found that the CT genotype of the SNP rs3957356 in *GSTA1* increases the risk of severe ARD by approximately 6-fold, with low certainty of evidence.

Other SNPS associated with the development of mild and severe ARD in this systematic review are reported in **Table 1.**

Considering that these SNPs have presented low or considerably low certainty of evidence of association with ARD, further studies should be carried out to evaluate these SNPs to verify the existence of this association.

2.2 Association IN patients with head and neck CANCER

There is still no systematic review that summarizes the data on SNPs in the prediction of ARD in patients with head and neck cancer. Therefore, the evidence discussed here comes from a quick literature search.

The rs3755557 SNP in *GSK3β* in the allelic model was reported [62] to have a statistically significant association with the development of severe ARD, considered to be a manifestation of moist desquamation. This gene participates in a number of tissue repair and inflammation pathways [63]. Therefore, it is hypothesized that polymorphisms in this gene may be associated with loss of function in the pathways and decreased tissue repair [56].

Borchiellini et al. [64] demonstrated an association between the GG genotype of SNP rs2279744 in *MDM2* and a 1.23-fold increase in the risk of severe ARD. This gene is responsible for *TP53* degradation [65].

SNPs associated with severe ARD			**SNPs associated with mild ARD**		
Gene	**SNP**	**Genotype**	**Gene**	**SNP**	**Genotype**
Wild homozygote			**Wild homozygote**		
PTTG1	rs3811999	CC	*PTTG1*	rs2961952	GG
PTTG1	rs2961950	AA	*CD44*	rs8193	CC
MAD2L2	rs2294638	GG			
MAT1A	rs2282367	GG			
Heterozygous			**Heterozygous**		
GSTA1	rs3957356	CT	*PTTG1*	rs3811999	GG
CD44	rs8193	CT	*MAT1A*	rs2282367	CC
SH3GL1	rs243336	GC			
			Variant homozygote		
			OGG1	rs2075747	AA

Table 1.
Single-nucleotide polymorphisms (SNPs) associated with acute radiation dermatitis (ARD) in the study by Aguiar et al. [48].

XRCC1 plays an important role in DNA repair following base excision damage [66]. Nanda et al. [67] and Raturi et al. [68] found that polymorphic variants in *XRCC1* for the SNP encoded by rs1799782 increased the risk of developing severe ARD. Additionally, Li et al. [69] found that polymorphic variants in this gene for the SNP encoded by rs25487 also increased the risk of developing severe ARD.

3. Conclusion

Severe degrees of ARD may cause local pain and burning, in addition to having a major impact on patients' quality of life and body image. Methods capable of predicting the occurrence and severity of ARD could improve RT planning. In addition to clinical tumor data and baseline data on patient characteristics, such as exposure to risk factors for ARD, the assessment of SNPs that can predict ARD could assist in patient follow-up and allow personalized RT planning. The use of predictive radiotoxicity genetic assays will allow patients who are more resistant to RT to receive higher doses of treatment without causing serious damage to adjacent tissues. Additionally, patients with lower RT tolerability receive another type of treatment or a lower dose of RT.

Thus, early detection of ARD susceptibility can improve the quality of life of patients who may develop severe ARD and the costs associated with the management of this radiotoxicity in the health care system.

Despite the promising role of SNPs in predicting ARD, studies have yielded inconsistent results and are not sufficient to confirm a significant association. Further studies are needed to confirm this hypothesis. We suggest that genes that have already been reported to have a statistically significant association in at least one study should be investigated in future.

Acknowledgements

The authors acknowledge the Graduate Program in Health Sciences at the University of Brasília - Brazil (Programa de Pós-Graduação em Ciências da Saúde da Universidade de Brasília - Brasil) for funding the publication of this chapter.

Author details

Beatriz Regina Lima de Aguiar, Eliete Neves Silva Guerra
and Paula Elaine Diniz dos Reis*
University of Brasília, Brasília, Brazil

*Address all correspondence to: pauladiniz@unb.br

References

[1] De Ruysscher D, Niedermann G, Burnet NG, Siva S, Lee AWM, Hegi-Johnson F. Radiotherapy toxicity. Nature Reviews Disease Primers. 2019: 1-20. DOI: 10.1038/s41572-019-0064-5

[2] Thiagarajan A, Iyer NG. Genomics of radiation sensitivity in squamous cell carcinomas. Pharmacogenomics. 2019;**20**(6):457-466. DOI: 10.2217/pgs-2018-0154

[3] Aguiar BRL, Reis PED, Normando AGC, Dia SS, Ferreira EB, Guerra ENS. Radiogenômica: Uma estratégia personalizada para predição de toxicidades induzidas por radiação. In: Santos M, Correa TS, Faria LDBB, Siqueira GSM, Reis PED, Pinheiro RN (org.). Diretrizes Oncológicas. 2nd ed. São Paulo: Doctor Press; 2019. pp. 1-8

[4] Marta GN. Radiobiologia: princípios básicos aplicados à prática clínica. Diagnóstico e tratamento. 2014;**19**(1):45-47

[5] Silva LFO, Santos LB. Física Médica Aplicada à Radioterapia. In: Santos M, Correa TS, Faria LDBB, Siqueira GSM, Reis PED, Pinheiro RN (org.). Diretrizes Oncológicas. 2nd ed. São Paulo: Doctor Press; 2018. pp. 591-606

[6] Suntharalingam N, Podgorsak EB, Hendry JH. Basic radiobiology. In: Podgorsak EB, editor. Radiation Oncology Physics: A Handbook for Teachers and Students. Vienna: International Atomic Energy Agency; 2005. pp. 485-504

[7] Mozdarani H, Salimi M, Bakhtari N. Inherent radiosensitivity and its impact on breast cancer chemo-radiotherapy. International Journal of Radiation Research. 2017;**15**(4):325-341. DOI: 10.18869/acadpub.ijrr.15.4.325

[8] Sia J, Szmyd R, Hau E, Gee HE. Molecular mechanisms of radiation-induced Cancer cell death: A primer. Frontiers in Cell and Development Biology. 2020;**8**:41. DOI: 10.3389/fcell.2020.00041

[9] Guo Z, Shu Y, Zhou H, Zhang W, Wang H. Radiogenomics helps to achieve personalized therapy by evaluating patient responses to radiation treatment. Carcinogenesis. 2015;**36**(3):307-317. DOI: 10.1093/carcin/bgv007

[10] Morton LM, Ricks-Santi L, West CML, Rosenstein BS. Radiogenomic predictors of adverse effects following charged particle therapy. International Journal of Particle Therapy. 2018;**5**(1):103-113. DOI: 10.14338/IJPT-18-00009.1

[11] Pawlik TM, Keyomarsi K. Role of cell cycle in mediating sensitivity to radiotherapy. International Journal of Radiaton Oncology. 2004;**59**(4):928-942. DOI: 10.1016/j.ijrobp.2004.03.005

[12] Pavlopoulou A, Bagos PG, Koutsandrea V, Georgakilas AG. Molecular determinants of radiosensitivity in normal and tumor tissue: A bioinformatic approach. Cancer Letters. 2017;**403**:37-47. DOI: 10.1016/j.canlet.2017.05.023

[13] Robijns J, Laubach HJ. Acute and chronic radiodermatitis clinical signs, pathophysiology, risk factors and management options. Journal of the Egyptian Women's Dermatologic Society. 2018;**15**(1):2-9. DOI: 10.1097/01.EWX.0000529960.52517.4c

[14] Rosenthal A, Israilevich R, Moy R. Management of acute radiation dermatitis: A review of the literature

and proposal for treatment algorithm. American Academy of Dermatology. 2019;**81**(2):558-567. DOI: 10.1016/j.jaad.2019.02.047

[15] Bontempo PSM, Meneses AG, Ciol M, Simino GPR, Ferreira EB, Reis PED. Acute radiodermatitis in cancer patients: Incidence and severity estimates. Revista da Escola de Enfermagem da USP. 2021;**55**:e03676. DOI: 10.1590/S1980- 220X2019021703676

[16] Iacovelli NA, Torrente Y, Ciuffreda A, Guardamagna VA, Gentili M, Giacomelli L, et al. Topical treatment of radiation-induced dermatitis: Current issues and potential solutions. Drugs Context. 2020;**2020**(9):4-7. DOI: 10.7573%2Fdic.2020-4-7

[17] Reis PED, Ferreira EB, Bontempo PSM. Radiodermatites: Prevenção e tratamento. In: Santos M, Correa TS, Faria LDBB, Siqueira GSM, Reis PED, Pinheiro RN (org.). Diretrizes Oncológicas. 2nd ed. São Paulo: Doctor Press; 2019. pp. 683-692

[18] Kole AJ, Kole L, Moran MS. Acute radiation dermatitis in breast cancer patients: Challenges and solutions. Breast Cancer-Targets and Therapy. 2017;**9**:313-323. DOI: 10.2147/BCTT.S109763

[19] CTCAE. Common Terminology Criteria for Adverse Events. Version 5.0. U.S Department of Health and Human Services; National Institutes of Health; National Cancer Institute; 2017 Available from: https://ctep.cancer.gov/protocoldevelopment/electronic_applications/docs/ctcae_v5_quick_reference_5x7.pdf

[20] Cox JD, Stetz J, Pajak TF. Toxicity criteria of the radiation therapy oncology group (RTOG) and the European Organization for Research and Treatment of Cancer (EORTC). International Journal of Radiation Oncology, Biology, Physics. 1995;**31**(5):1341-1346. DOI: 10.1016/0360-3016(95)00060-c

[21] Gosselin T, Ginex PK, Backler C, Bruce SD, Hutton A, Marquez CM, et al. ONS guidelines™ for Cancer treatment-related Radiodermatitis. Oncology Nursing Forum. 2020;**47**(6):654-670. DOI: 10.1188/20.onf.654-670

[22] Ferreira EB, Vasques CI, Gadia R, Chan RJ, Guerra ENS, Mezzomo LA, et al. Topical interventions to prevent acute radiation dermatitis in head and neck cancer patients: A systematic review. Supportive Care in Cancer. 2017;**25**(3):1001-1011. DOI: 10.1007/s00520-016-3521-7

[23] Costa CC, Lyra JS, Nakamura RA, Sousa CM. Radiodermatitis: Analysis of predictive factors in breast Cancer patients. Revista Brasileira de Cancerologia. 2019;**65**(1):e-05275. DOI: 10.32635/2176-9745.RBC.2019 v65n1.275

[24] Barnett GC, Kerns SL, Noble DJ, Dunning AM, West CM, Burnet NG. Incorporating genetic biomarkers into predictive models of Normal tissue toxicity. Clinical Oncology (Royal College of Radiologists). 2015;**27**(10):579-587. DOI: 10.1016/j.clon.2015.06.013

[25] Safwat A, Bentzen SM, Turesson I, Hendry JH. Deterministic rather than stochastic factors explain most of the variation in the expression of skin telangiectasia after radiotherapy. International Journal of Radiation Oncology, Biology, Physics. 2002;**52**(1):198-204. DOI: 10.1016/s0360-3016(01)02690-6

[26] Pollard JM, Gatti RA. Clinical radiation sensitivity with DNA repair

disorders: An overview. International Journal of Radiation Oncology, Biology, Physics. 2009;**74**(5):1323-1331. DOI: 10.1016/j.ijrobp.2009.02.057

[27] Brothwell MRS, West CM, Dunning AM, Burnet NG, Barnett GC. Radiogenomics in the era of advanced radiotherapy. Clinical Oncology (Royal College of Radiologists). 2019;**31**(5):319-325. DOI: 10.1016/j.clon.2019.02.006

[28] Kang J, Coates JT, Strawderman RL, Rosenstein BS, Kerns SL. Genomics models in radiotherapy: From mechanistic to machine learning. Medical Physics. 2020;**47**(5):e203-e217. DOI: 10.1002/mp.13751

[29] Meehan J, Gray M, Martínez-Pérez C, Kay C, Pang LY, Fraser JA, et al. Precision medicine and the role of biomarkers of radiotherapy response in breast Cancer. Frontiers in Oncology. 2020;**10**:628. DOI: 10.3389%2Ffonc.2020.00628

[30] West C, Rosenstein BS, Alsner J, Azria D, Barnett G, Begg A, et al. Establishment of a Radiogenomics consortium. International Journal of Radiation Oncology, Biology, Physics. 2010;**76**(5):1295-1296. DOI: 10.1016/j.ijrobp.2009.12.017

[31] National Cancer Institute. Epidemiology and Genomics Research Program. 2019. Available from: https://epi.grants.cancer.gov/radiogenomics/. [Accessed: August 17, 2021]

[32] Hall WA, Bergom C, Thompson RF, Torres-Roca JF, Weidhaas J, Feng FY, et al. Precision oncology and Genomically guided radiation therapy: A report from the American Society for Radiation Oncology/American Association of Physicists in Medicine/National Cancer Institute precision medicine conference. International Journal of Radiation Oncology. 2017;**101**(2):274-284. DOI: 10.1016/j.ijrobp.2017.05.044 146

[33] Story MD, Durante M. Radiogenomics. Medical Physics. 2018;**45**(11):1111-1112. DOI: 10.1002/mp.13064

[34] Wang MH, Cordell HJ, Steen KV. Statistical methods for genome-wide association studies. Seminars in Cancer Biology. 2019;**55**:53-60. DOI: 10.1016/j.semcancer.2018.04.008

[35] Vallejos-Vidal E, Reyes-Cerpa S, Rivas-Pardo JA, Maisey K, Yáñez JM, Valenzuela H, et al. Single-nucleotide polymorphisms (SNP) mining and their effect on the tridimensional protein structure prediction in a set of immunity related expressed sequence tags (EST) in Atlantic Salmon (Salmo salar). Frontiers in Genetics. 2020;**10**:1406. DOI: 10.3389/fgene.2019.01406

[36] Karki R, Pandya D, Elston RC, Ferlini C. Defining "mutation" and "polymorphism" in the era of personal genomics. BMC Medical Genomics. 2015;**8**:37. DOI: 10.1186%2Fs12920-015-0115-z

[37] Al-Koofee DAF, Mubarak SMH. Genetic polymorphisms. In: Çalışkan M, Erol O, Öz GC, editors. The Recent Topics in Genetic Polymorphisms. London: IntechOpen; 2019. DOI: 10.5772/intechopen.88063

[38] Huang T, Shu Y, Cai YD. Genetic differences among ethnic groups. BMC Genomics. 2015;**16**:1093. DOI: 10.1186%2Fs12864-015-2328-0

[39] Rosenstein BS. Radiogenomics: Identification of genomic predictors for radiation toxicity. Seminars in Radiation Oncology. 2017;**27**(4):300-309. DOI: 10.1016%2Fj.semradonc.2017.04.005

[40] 1000 Genomes Project Consortium, Auton A, Brooks LD, Durbin RM, Garrison EP, Kang HM, et al. A global reference for human genetic variation. Nature. 2015;**526**(7571):68-74. DOI: 10.1038/nature15393

[41] Condit CM, Achter PJ, Lauer I, Sefcovic E. The changing meanings of "mutation:" a contextualized study of public discourse. Human Mutation. 2002;**19**:69-75. DOI: 10.1002/humu.10023

[42] Richards S, Aziz N, Bale S, Bick D, Das S, Gastier-Foster J. Standards and guidelines for the interpretation of sequence variants: A joint consensus recommendation of the American College of Medical Genetics and Genomics and the Association for Molecular Pathology. Genetics in Medicine. 2015;**17**(5):405-424. DOI: 10.1038%2Fgim.2015.30

[43] Alberts B et al. . In: 6th ed., editor. Biologia molecular da célula. Artmed: Porto Alegre; 2017. p. 471

[44] Ahmad T, Valentovic MA, Rankin GO. Effects of cytochrome P450 single nucleotide polymorphisms on methadone metabolism and pharmacodynamics. 147. Biochemical Pharmacology. 2018;**153**:196-204. DOI: 10.1016/j.bcp.2018.02.020

[45] Turchetto-Zolet AC, Turchetto C, Guzman F, Silva-Arias GA, Sperb-Ludwig F, Veto NM. Polimorfismo de Nucleotídeo único (SNP): metodologias de identificação, análise e aplicações. In: Turchetto-Zolet AC, Turchetto C, Zanella CM, Passaia G (Org.). Marcadores Moleculares na Era genômica: Metodologias e Aplicações. Ribeirão Preto: Sociedade Brasileira de Genética; 2017. pp. 133-179

[46] Huang A, Glick SA. Genetic susceptibility to cutaneous radiation injury. Archives of Dermatological Research. 2017;**1**:10. DOI: 10.1007/s00403-016-1702-3

[47] Seibold P, Behrens S, Schmezer P, West CM, Popanda O, Chang-Claude J. XRCC1 polymorphism associated with late toxicity after radiation therapy in breast Cancer patients. International Journal of Radiation Oncology. 2015;**92**(5):1084-1092. DOI: 10.1016/j.ijrobp.2015.04.011

[48] Aguiar BRL, Ferreira EB, Normando AGC, Mazzeu JF, Assad DX, Guerra ENS, et al. Single nucleotide polymorphisms to predict acute radiation dermatitis in breast cancer patients: A systematic review and meta-analysis. Critical Reviews in Oncology/Hematology. 2022;**173**:103651. DOI: 10.1016/j.critrevonc.2022.103651

[49] Mumbrekar KD, Sadashiva SRB, Kabekkodu SP, Fernandes DJ, Vadhiraja BM, Suga T, et al. Genetic variants in CD44 and MAT1A confer susceptibility to acute skin reaction in breast Cancer patients undergoing radiation therapy. International Journal of Radiation Oncology Biology Physics. 2017;**97**(1):118-127. DOI: 10.1016/j.ijrobp.2016.09.017

[50] Suga TM, Ishikawa A, Kohda M, Otsuka Y, Yamada S, Yamamoto N, et al. Haplotype-based analysis of genes associated with risk of adverse skin reactions after radiotherapy in breast cancer patients. International Journal of Radiation Oncology, Biology, Physics. 2007;**69**(3):685-693. DOI: 10.1016/j.ijrobp.2007.06.021

[51] Chen C, Zhao S, Karnad A, Freeman JW. The biology and role of CD44 in cancer progression: Therapeutic implications. Journal of Hematology & Oncology. 2018;**11**(1):64. DOI: 10.1186%2Fs13045-018-0605-5

[52] Mokhtarian R, Tabatabaeian H, Saadatmand P, Azadeh M, Balmeh N, Yakhchali B, et al. CD44 gene rs8193 C allele is significantly enriched in gastric Cancer patients. Cell Journal. 2020;**21**(4):451-458. DOI: 10.22074%2Fcellj.2020.6389

[53] Deng Y, Chen ZJ, Lan F, He QT, Chen SY, Du YF, et al. Association of CD44 polymorphisms and susceptibility to HBV-related hepatocellular carcinoma in the Chinese population. Journal of Clinical Laboratory Analysis. 2019;**33**(8):e22977. DOI: 10.1002/jcla.22977

[54] Al-Othman N, Alhendi A, Ihbaisha M, Barahmeh M, Alqaraleh M, Al-Momany BZ. Role of CD44 in breast cancer. Breast Disease. 2020;**39**(1):1-13. DOI: 10.3233/bd-190409

[55] Lin X, You X, Cao X, Pan S. Association of Single-Nucleotide Polymorphisms of CD44 gene with susceptibility to breast Cancer in Chinese women. Medical Science Monitor. 2018;**24**:3077-3083. DOI: 10.12659%2FMSM.907422

[56] Govindaraju P, Todd L, Shetye S, Monslow J, Puré E. CD44-dependent inflammation, fibrogenesis, and collagenolysis regulates extracellular matrix remodeling and tensile strength during cutaneous wound healing. Matrix Biology. 2019;**75-76**:314-330. DOI: 10.1016/j.matbio.2018.06.004

[57] Murray RJS, Tanteles GA, Mills J, Perry A, Peat I, Osman A, et al. Association between single nucleotide polymorphisms in the DNA repair gene LIG3 and acute adverse skin reactions following radiotherapy. Radiotherapy and Oncology. 2011;**99**:231-234. DOI: 10.1016/j.radonc.2011.05.007

[58] Hua RX, Zhuo Z, Zhu J, Zhang SD, Xue WQ, Li X, et al. LIG3 gene polymorphisms and risk of gastric cancer in a southern Chinese population. Gene. 2019;**705**:90-94. DOI: 10.1016/j.gene.2019.04.072

[59] Condorelli AG, El Hachem M, Zambruno G, Nystrom A, Candi E, Castiglia D. Notch-ing up knowledge on molecular mechanisms of skin fibrosis: Focus on the multifaceted notch signalling pathway. Journal of Biomedical Science. 2021;**28**(1):36. DOI: 10.1186/s12929-021-00732-8

[60] Barnett GC, Elliott RM, Alsner J, Andreassen CN, Abdelhay O, Burnet NG, et al. Individual patient data meta-analysis shows no association between the SNP rs1800469 in TGFB and late radiotherapy toxicity. Radiotherapy and Oncology. 2012;**105**(3):289-295. DOI: 10.1016/j.radonc.2012.10.017

[61] Rattay T, Talbot CJ. Finding the genetic determinants of adverse reactions to radiotherapy. Clinical Oncology (Royal College of Radiologists). 2014;**26**(5):301-308. DOI: 10.1016/j.clon.2014.02.001

[62] Yu J, Huang Y, Liu L, Wang J, Yin J, Huang L, et al. Genetic polymorphisms of Wnt/β-catenin pathway genes are associated with the efficacy and toxicities of radiotherapy in patients with nasopharyngeal carcinoma. Oncotarget. 2016;**7**(50):82528-82537. DOI: 10.18632%2Foncotarget.12754

[63] Lin J, Song T, Li C, Mao W. GSK-3β in DNA repair, apoptosis, and resistance of chemotherapy, radiotherapy of cancer. Biochimica et Biophysica Acta - Molecular Cell Research. 2020;**1867**(5):118659. DOI: 10.1016/j.bbamcr.2020.118659

[64] Borchiellini D, Etienne-Grimaldi MC, Bensadoun RJ, Benezery K, Dassonville O, Poissonnet G, et al. Candidate apoptotic and DNA repair

gene approach confirms involvement of ERCC1, ERCC5, TP53 and MDM2 in radiation-induced toxicity in head and neck cancer. Oral Oncology. 2017;**67**:70-76. DOI: 10.1016/j.oraloncology.2017.02.003

[65] Gupta A, Shah K, Oza MJ, Behl T. Reactivation of p53 gene by MDM2 inhibitors: A novel therapy for cancer treatment. Biomedicine & Pharmacotherapy. 2019;**109**:484-492. DOI: 10.1016/j.biopha.2018.10.155

[66] Moghaddam AS, Nazarzadeh M, Noroozi R, Darvish H, Mosavi JA. XRCC1 and OGG1 gene polymorphisms and breast Cancer: A systematic review of literature. Iranian Journal of Cancer Prevention. 2016;**9**(1):e3467. DOI: 10.17795/ijcp-3467

[67] Nanda SS, Gandhi AK, Rastogi M, Khurana R, Hadi R, Sahni K, et al. Evaluation of XRCC1 gene polymorphism as a biomarker in head and neck Cancer patients undergoing Chemoradiation therapy. International Journal of Radiation Oncology, Biology, Physics. 2018;**101**(3):593-601. DOI: 10.1016/j.ijrobp.2018.03.039

[68] Raturi V, Hojo H, Bhatt MLB, Suhel M, Wu CT, Bei Y, et al. Prospective evaluation of XRCC-1 Arg194Trp polymorphism as bio-predictor for clinical outcome in locally advanced laryngeal cancer undergoing cisplatin-based chemoradiation. Head & Neck. 2020;**42**(5):1045-1056. DOI: 10.1002/hed.26083

[69] Li H, You Y, Lin C, Zheng M, Hong C, Chen J, et al. XRCC1 codon 399Gln polymorphism is associated with radiotherapy-induced acute dermatitis and mucositis in nasopharyngeal carcinoma patients. Radiation Oncology. 2013;**8**:31. DOI: 10.1186/1748-717X-8-31

Chapter 4

Cervical Cancer

Eter Natelauri

Abstract

Cervical cancer is a worldwide public health problem. The leading cause of cervical cancer is persistent infection with high-risk human papillomavirus (HPV). Vaccines exist that protect against high-risk HPV types, and screening programs can detect signs of disease at an early stage, allowing for effective treatment and management of the condition. While being one of the most preventable and treatable forms of cancer, the mortality rate is high, especially in low- and middle-income countries. Early diagnoses, proper staging, and a multidisciplinary approach is the cornerstone of disease management. Surgical treatment, radiation therapy, chemotherapy, immune therapy, and supportive and palliative care are all essential parts of the complex treatment. A simple hysterectomy or brachytherapy for early-stage cervical cancer results in a 5-year OS of more than 98%. For selected patients, radical trachelectomy represents a fertility-sparing treatment option. Radiotherapy (RT), with or without cisplatin-based concurrent chemotherapy after radical or modified radical hysterectomy, is recommended for patients with intermediate- or high-risk features. RT, including brachytherapy plus concurrent chemotherapy, is the treatment of choice for patients with locally advanced disease. Irradiation often provides excellent short-term relief of pain and bleeding, particularly in patients with no history of prior RT.

Keywords: cervical cancer, HPV, staging, FIGO, hysterectomy, radiotherapy, brachytherapy, adjuvant radiotherapy

1. Introduction

According to WHO, in 2020, an estimated 604,000 females were diagnosed with cervical cancer worldwide, and about 342,000 females died from the disease [1]. Every year in the United States, about 13,000 new cases of cervical cancer are diagnosed, and about 4000 women die of cervix cancer. Hispanic females have the highest rates of developing cervical cancer, and Black females have the highest rates of dying from cervical cancer [2]. The highest incidences occur in populations with a high prevalence of human papillomavirus (HPV) infection and inadequate screening rates. The mortality rates for cervical cancer range from less than 2 per 100,000 in western Asia, Western Europe, and Australia to more than 20 per 100,000 in central America, Melanesia, and the majority of Africa due to these factors, plus variances in access to effective therapies [3]. Most covariables traditionally associated with an increased risk of cervical cancer appear to be surrogates for sexually transmitted HPV infection. The results of tumor DNA analysis show that practically all squamous or adenocarcinoma of the cervix cases integrate DNA from at least one of multiple high-risk HPV subtypes. HPV16, HPV18, HPV31, HPV33, and HPV45 are high-risk subtypes; the most prevalent are HPV16 and HPV18, which account for around 70% of cervical malignancies. Risk factors for cervix cancer and its intraepithelial precursors include early coitus, multiple sexual partners, and a history of other sexually transmitted infections [4]. Although some researchers have observed a link between cervical cancer with continued oral contraceptive usage, various confounding risk factors and changes in diagnostic criteria make it challenging to demonstrate a causal relationship [5].

2. Anatomy and pathology

The cervix is the lower portion of the uterus that joins the corpus to the vagina (from the Latin collar, "neck"). The exocervix, also referred to as the ectocervix, protrudes into the top vagina and is protected with squamous epithelium. The canal that connects to the endometrial hollow space is the endocervix. It has a single layer of mucinous columnar cells and longitudinal mucosal ridges consisting of fibrovascular cores. The macroscopic intersection of the exocervix and endocervix is known as the external os. The microscopic connection of the mucous and squamous, columnar epithelia is called the squamocolumnar junction. The isthmus also referred to as the decreased uterine phase, is the area between the endocervix and the endometrial hollow space [6].

The transformation sector is the region among the most distal squamocolumnar juncture and the external os. This quarter's immature squamous epithelium exhibits progressive nuclear maturation and increases the glycogen-loose cytoplasm closer to the surface. Colposcopy has a thin white membrane that thickens and turns white as the squamous epithelium grows. As cells collect glycogen, they become indistinguishable from the typical exocervical squamous epithelium. The transformation zone is where cervical squamous cancers mainly develop [6]. The classification of cervical epithelial alterations according to their histological characteristics differentiates groups of women based on the state of cellular maturation, and the thickness of the affected area in the squamous epithelium is presented in **Table 1**.

The Bethesda system divides cytological specimens into two main groups, low-grade squamous intraepithelial lesions (LSILs) and high-grade squamous intraepithelial lesions (HSILs) [7]. LSILs are characterized by modifications in mature squamous cells (superficial or intermediate) because of HPV, and the morphological modifications are identical to slight dysplasia or low-grade intraepithelial lesion (NIC1). The possibility of growing a high-grade intraepithelial lesion or most cancers over 5 years is 18% [8]. HSILs are characterized by losing the nucleus-to-cytoplasm ratio in the tiniest, maximum juvenile squamous cells (para-basal). This is the primary indicator of the pathology. The presence of NIC2, NIC3, and in situ most cancers in the histological section is all additives of an HSIL analysis in cytology. A NIC2 or NIC3 biopsy is carried out on most patients who have been diagnosed with HSIL [9]. Squamous cell carcinoma is an epithelial invasive tumor constructed from differentiated squamous cells. The Bethesda system does not subdivide squamous cell carcinoma in the same manner as the WHO category system. Keratinizing, non-keratinizing, papillary, basaloid, warty, squamous-transitional, and lymphoepithelial are the classifications used by the WHO (**Table 2**). This is because morphological developments cannot be outstanding through cytology information. Atypical glandular cells (AHCs) refer to abnormalities in the glandular epithelium that go beyond

Specimen adequacy
Satisfactory for evaluation (*note presence/absence of endocervical/transformation zone component*)
Unsatisfactory for evaluation ... (*specify reason*). Specimen rejected/not processed (*specify reason*)
Specimen processed and examined, but unsatisfactory for evaluation of epithelial abnormality because of (*specify reason*)
General categorization (*optional*)
Negative for intraepithelial lesion or malignancy epithelial cell abnormality
Other
Interpretation/result
Negative for intraepithelial lesion or malignancy
Organisms
Trichomonas vaginalis
Fungal organisms morphologically consistent with *Candida* species shift in flora suggestive of bacterial vaginosis
Bacteria morphologically consistent with *Actinomyces* species cellular changes consistent with herpes simplex virus
Other non-neoplastic findings (*optional to report; list not comprehensive*)
Reactive cellular changes associated with inflammation (includes typical repair) radiation
Intrauterine contraceptive device glandular cells status post hysterectomy atrophy
Epithelial cell abnormalities
Squamous cell
Atypical squamous cells (ASC) of undetermined significance (ASC-US) cannot exclude HSIL (ASC-H)
Low-grade squamous intraepithelial lesion (LSIL) encompassing: human papillomavirus/mild dysplasia/cervical intraepithelial neoplasia (CIN) 1
High-grade squamous intraepithelial lesion (HSIL) encompassing: moderate and severe dysplasia, carcinoma in situ; CIN 2 and CIN 3
Squamous cell carcinoma glandular cell
Atypical glandular cells (AGC) (*specify endocervical, endometrial, or not otherwise specified*)
Atypical glandular cells, favor neoplastic (*specify endocervical or not otherwise specified*)
Endocervical adenocarcinoma in situ (AIS) adenocarcinoma
Other (*List not comprehensive*)
Endometrial cells in a woman S40 years of age

Table 1.
The 2001 Bethesda System (Abridged).

Squamous epithelial tumors
- Mimics of squamous precursor lesions
  - Squamous metaplasia
  - Atrophy of the uterine cervix
- Squamous cell tumors and precursors
  - Condyloma acuminatum
  - Squamous intraepithelial lesions of the uterine cervix
  - Squamous cell carcinoma, HPV associated, of the uterine cervix
  - Squamous cell carcinoma, HPV independent, of the uterine cervix
  - Squamous cell carcinoma, NOS of the uterine cervix

Glandular tumors and precursors
- Benign glandular lesions
  - Endocervical polyp
  - Müllerian papilloma of the uterine cervix
  - Nabothian cyst
  - Tunnel clusters
  - Microglandular hyperplasia
  - Lobular endocervical glandular hyperplasia
  - Diffuse laminar endocervical hyperplasia
  - Mesonephric remnants and hyperplasia
  - Arias Stella reaction of the uterine cervix
  - Endocervicosis of the uterine cervix

- Tuboendometrioid metaplasia
- Ectopic prostate tissue
- Adenocarcinomas
    - Adenocarcinoma in situ, HPV associated, of the uterine cervix
    - Adenocarcinoma, HPV associated, of the uterine cervix
    - Adenocarcinoma in situ, HPV independent, of the uterine cervix
    - Adenocarcinoma, HPV independent, gastric type, of the uterine cervix
    - Adenocarcinoma, HPV independent, clear cell type, of the uterine cervix
    - Adenocarcinoma, HPV independent, mesonephric type, of the uterine cervix
    - Other adenocarcinomas of the uterine cervix
- Other epithelial tumors
    - Carcinosarcoma of the uterine cervix
    - Adenosquamous and mucoepidermoid carcinomas of the uterine cervix
    - Adenoid basal carcinoma of the uterine cervix
    - Carcinoma of the uterine cervix, unclassifiable
- Mixed epithelial and mesenchymal tumors
    - Adenomyoma of the uterine cervix
    - Adenosarcoma of the uterine cervix
- Germ cell tumors
    - Germ cell tumors of the uterine cervix

Table 2.
The World Health Organization classification of tumors cervix, 5th edition (2020).

reactive changes but are insufficient to classify them as adenocarcinoma. The morphological entities that advise this prognosis may be benign or malignant. The benign conditions include endocervical and endometrial polyps, endometriosis, endocervical microcystic hyperplasia, adenosis, lively and lower uterine phase brushings, tubal metaplasia, and Arias-Stella phenomenon. Malignant situations include high-grade intraepithelial lesions with glandular penetration, in situ adenocarcinoma, and invasive adenocarcinoma [10].

Other pathological types of cervical cancer include endometrioid adenocarcinoma, clear cell adenocarcinoma, adenosquamous carcinoma, adenoid cystic carcinoma, adenoid basal cell carcinoma, small cell carcinoma, neuroendocrine carcinoma, and undifferentiated carcinoma.

Squamous cell carcinomas arise between 80 and 90% of all cervical cancers. Those designations no longer correspond correctly with analysis, despite the reality that squamous neoplasms are often sub-classified as large-cell keratinizing, huge-cellular no keratinizing, or small-cellular carcinomas [11]. It is estimated that between 10 and 20% of women may develop primary cervical adenocarcinoma throughout their lifetimes, although the incidence of this cancer appears to be on the rise, particularly in younger females [12].

3. Pathways of spread

Most cervical cancers start where the epithelium of the endocervix, frequently columnar, meets the epithelium of the ectocervix, which is especially squamous. As soon as a tumor has broken through the basement membrane, it can either move straight into the cervical stroma or use blood vessels to reach it. Invasive tumors can start as exophytic growths that stick out of the cervix into the vagina or endocervical lesions, which could purpose the cervix to grow very massive, although the ectocervix seems regular. From the cervix, the tumor can spread to the lower part of the uterus, the vagina, the extensive ligaments in which it could block the ureter, or the uterosacral ligaments, also causing blockage of the ureter. During a pelvic exam, massive tumors may additionally seem fixed. However, an actual invasion of the muscle tissues of the pelvic wall is uncommon. Even though there may be a thin layer of fascia and cell connective tissue between the cervix and the bladder, giant bladder involvement is uncommon in less than 5% of instances. The tumor may additionally spread back to the rectum. However, rectal mucosal involvement at the time of diagnosis is rare. The mucosal, muscular, and serosal layers of the cervix are well-drained by three anastomosing plexuses of lymphatics [13]. The cardinal ligament has a supra-ureteral pathway, and the uterosacral ligament has a dorsal pathway toward the rectal pillars. The vesicouterine ligament drains the upper vagina and bladder and has no lymphatic drainage from the cervix [14]. Three major lymphatic collecting trunks leave the uterine isthmus laterally. The upper branches follow the uterine artery from the anterior and lateral cervix, the intermediate branches drain to the deeper hypogastric (obturator) nodes, and the lowest branches drain posteriorly to the inferior and superior gluteal, common iliac, presacral, and subaortic lymph nodes.

Tumor stage, tumor size, histologic subtype, depth of invasion (DOI), and the existence of lymph vascular space invasion (LVSI) are all associated with the risk of pelvic and para-aortic node involvement. Almost all data on regional nodal metastases come from subjects that had lymphadenectomy as part of radical surgeries earlier than radiation therapy, and those numbers can range significantly. Studies have reported a 15–20% positivity rate for pelvic nodes and 1–5% for para-aortic nodes of patients with stage I disease who underwent radical hysterectomy for their treatment. Depending on many factors, including a physical exam and risk factors, the proportion of patients with positive nodes may be higher than 50% in those with more advanced diseases [15].

Hematogenous metastases are infrequent at diagnosis, and two-thirds of relapsed patients had pelvic disease. Relapses often involve distant metastases. Fagundes et al. found 10-year actuarial rates for distant metastases of 16%, 31%, 26%, and 39% for FIGO stages IB, IIA, IIB, and III radiotherapy (RT) patients, respectively [16]. If pelvic sickness is the first website of relapse, a systematic radiological assessment might not be executed, underestimating these. Lung metastases were the most commonplace extra pelvic region. Although the lumbar spine is a not unusual supply of skeletal metastasis, computed tomography (CT) indicates that women who appear to have isolated metastases may additionally rather have direct tumor extension from PA nodal disease [17].

4. Staging

The cervix was the first organ for which The International Federation of Gynecology and Obstetrics (FIGO) established a system for only clinical staging in 1958. Thereafter, to document the presence or absence of nodes and distant metastases, a pathological TNM staging system was developed and implemented. The FIGO Committee of Gynecological Oncology updated the staging system in 2018 so that clinical, radiological, or pathological evidence may be used to designate the stage (**Table 3**).

Clinical examination and physical evaluation initiate staging. FIGO 2018 staging allows ultrasonography, CT, MRI, and PET to offer further information about tumor size, nodal status, and local or systemic metastasis [18]. MRI is helpful for primary

Stage	Description
I	The carcinoma is strictly confined to the cervix (extension to the uterine corpus should be disregarded)
IA	Invasive carcinoma that can be diagnosed only by microscopy, with maximum depth of invasion ≤5 mm[a]
IA1	Measured stromal invasion ≤3 mm in depth
IA2	Measured stromal invasion >3 and ≤5 mm in depth
IB	Invasive carcinoma with measured deepest invasion >5 mm (greater than Stage IA); lesion limited to the cervix uteri with size measured by maximum tumor diameter[b]
IB1	Invasive carcinoma >5 mm depth of stromal invasion and ≤2 cm in greatest dimension
IB2	Invasive carcinoma >2 and ≤4 cm in greatest dimension
IB3	Invasive carcinoma >4 cm in greatest dimension
II	The carcinoma invades beyond the uterus, but has not extended onto the lower third of the vagina or to the pelvic wall
IIA	Involvement limited to the upper two-thirds of the vagina without parametrial involvement
IIA1	Invasive carcinoma ≤4 cm in greatest dimension
IIA2	Invasive carcinoma >4 cm in greatest dimension
IIB	With parametrial involvement but not up to the pelvic wall
III	The carcinoma involves the lower third of the vagina and/or extends to the pelvic wall and/or causes hydronephrosis or nonfunctioning kidney and/or involves pelvic and/or para-aortic lymph nodes
IIIA	The carcinoma involves the lower third of the vagina, with no extension to the pelvic wall
IIIB	Extension to the pelvic wall and/or hydronephrosis or nonfunctioning kidney (unless known to be due to another cause)
IIIC	Involvement of pelvic and/or para-aortic lymph nodes (including micrometastases)[c], irrespective of tumor size and extent (with r and p notations)[d]
IIIC1	Pelvic lymph node metastasis only
IIIC2	Para-aortic lymph node metastasis
IV	The carcinoma has extended beyond the true pelvis or has involved (biopsy proven) the mucosa of the bladder or rectum. A bullous edema, as such, does not permit a case to be allotted to Stage IV
IVA	Spread of the growth to adjacent pelvic organs
IVB	Spread to distant organs

[a]Imaging and pathology can be used, where available, to supplement clinical findings with respect to tumor size and extent, in all stages. Pathological findings supersede imaging and clinical findings.[b]The involvement of vascular/lymphatic spaces should not change the staging. The lateral extent of the lesion is no longer considered.[c]Isolated tumor cells do not change the stage but their presence should be recorded.[d]Adding notation of r (imaging) and p (pathology) to indicate the findings that are used to allocate the case to Stage IIIC. For example, if imaging indicates pelvic lymph node metastasis, the stage allocation would be Stage IIIC1r; if confirmed by pathological findings, it would be Stage IIIC1p. The type of imaging modality or pathology technique used should always be documented. When in doubt, the lower staging should be assigned.

Table 3.
FIGO staging of cancer of the cervix uteri (2018).

cancers beyond 10 mm. In experienced hands, ultrasonography provides high diagnostic preciseness. For future evaluation, note the staging modality. Imaging can provide new prognostic indicators to assist in choosing the best therapy. PET-CT is more accurate than CT and MRI (4–15% false-negative results) at detecting nodal metastases above 10 mm.

5. Work up

History and physical: Presentation may include postcoital bleeding, irregular or heavy vaginal bleeding, vaginal discharge, and lower back or pelvic pain. It may be asymptomatic and detected during the routine gynecologic examination.

Conduct complete pelvic examination, including bimanual examination and placement of fiducial markers at the caudal extent of vaginal disease. The patient should be positioned in a dorsal lithotomy during the examination. The rectovaginal exam gives information about parametrial extension and infiltration.

Labs: CBC, CMP, and LFTs. Consider HIV testing and pregnancy test.

Procedures/biopsy: Cervical biopsy and cone biopsy as indicated. For advanced stages (stage ≥IB2), consider examination under anesthesia, cystoscopy, and/or proctoscopy as indicated.

Pathology reports should always include information about a stromal invasion, lymph vascular space invasion (LVSI), sizes of the primary tumor, characteristics of margins and distance from the margins, parametrial invasion, number of dissected nodes, and number of positive nodes. The location of positive nodes is also essential, especially when an extranodal extension (ENE) is present.

Imaging: PET/CT. Pelvic MRI with intravaginal water-based gel. Chest imaging with a chest X-ray or CT chest.

6. Treatment

As a result of the fact that those with cervical cancer typically present with a mass that is clinically limited to the pelvis, achieving locoregional disease control is the fundamental obstacle that must be overcome throughout therapy [19]. Patients with an illness limited to a specific area see unprecedented rates of cure after receiving individualized treatment depending on the features of their tumors (**Table 4**).

Microinvasive cancers invading less than 3 mm (stage IA1) are treated with conservative surgery, including excisional conization or extra fascial hysterectomy. Early-stage invasive tumors, meaning stage IA2 and IB1 and some small stage IIA1, are treated with radical or modified radical hysterectomy, radical trachelectomy (when fertility preservation is needed/desired), or RT. Selected patients with centrally recurring illness following radical dose RT may have radical pelvic exenteration; isolated pelvic recurrence after hysterectomy is often treated with RT.

The standard of care for stage IA1 patients is usually cervical conization or total (Type I) hysterectomy. Because less aggressive tumors have less than a 1% chance of developing pelvic lymph node metastases, pelvic lymph node dissection is often not recommended for patients with these tumors. Lymph node metastases are possible in 5% of patients whose tumors extend 3–5 mm into the stroma (FIGO stage IA2) [20]. For such patients, a modified radical (type II) hysterectomy should be performed along with bilateral pelvic lymphadenectomy. The modified radical hysterectomy is a less invasive surgery than the traditional radical hysterectomy (type III). Patients with stages IA2 to IB1 cervical cancer who have low-risk factors are being considered for potential fertility-sparing surgery. Women treated with radical hysterectomy or

Stage (FIGO 2009)	Treatment	5-year OS
IA1 (no lymphovascular space invasion [LVSI])	Extra fascial hysterectomy or modified radical hysterectomy (RH) ➜ evaluate risk factors that may require adjuvant treatment *If fertility-sparing: Conization with negative margins*	>98%
IA1 (LVSI+) and IA2	Modified RH + pelvic lymph node dissection (PLND) ➜ evaluate risk factors that may require adjuvant treatment OR Pelvic RT + brachytherapy *If fertility sparing: Cone biopsy or radical trachelectomy + PLND*	≥95%
IB1/smaller IIA1	RH + PLND ± para-aortic sampling ➜ evaluate risk factors that may require adjuvant treatment OR pelvic RT + brachytherapy OR chemoRT (pelvic RT + cisplatin) + brachytherapy *If fertility sparing is desired: Radical trachelectomy + PLND may be considered for IB1*	~90%
IB2/larger IIA1/IIA2	ChemoRT (pelvic RT + cisplatin) + brachytherapy	80–85%
IIB		70–75%
III		~50%
IVA	ChemoRT (pelvic RT + cisplatin) + brachytherapy; exenteration in selected cases	15–25%
IVB, limited (oligometastatic disease)	ChemoRT (pelvic RT + cisplatin) + brachytherapy ± metastasectomy ±SBRT/SRT/SRS	5–15%
IVB	Chemotherapy; palliative radiotherapy	~0%

Table 4.
Primary therapy and survival by disease extenta.

radical trachelectomy tend to have comparable outcomes, and a considerable percentage of patients treated with radical trachelectomy report successful pregnancies [21]. Although surgery is the treatment of choice for in situ and microinvasive cancer, people with significant medical conditions or other contraindications to surgery can be effectively treated with radiation therapy. Depending on the depth of invasion, these early lesions are treated with brachytherapy or brachytherapy combined with external RT, with cure rates over 95% [22].

Early-stage IB and IIA cervical carcinomas may be efficaciously handled with a combination of external-beam radiation therapy (EBRT) and brachytherapy or with radical hysterectomy and bilateral pelvic lymphadenectomy. Patients undergoing radical hysterectomy high-risk disease may gain from postoperative RT or chemoradiation [23]. Overall, disease-specific survival rates for individuals with stage IB cervical cancer treated with surgery or radiation are typically in the 80–90% range. The decision of therapy for patients with stage IB1 squamous carcinomas depends primarily on patient desire, risks associated with general anesthesia and surgery, physician preference, and an awareness of the nature and occurrence of problems with hysterectomy and radiation. Some surgeons have also advocated radical hysterectomy as the first line of therapy for individuals with stage IB2 tumors [24, 25]. Then again, patients with tumors larger than 4 cm in diameter usually have enough risk factors to necessitate adjuvant EBRT or chemoradiation, increasing the treatment time and adverse events [23, 26]. As a result, many gynecologic and radiation oncologists claim that patients with stage IB2 carcinomas benefit from chemoradiation, although these two therapies have never been directly compared in a prospective trial.

Radiation therapy is the recommended main local therapy for the vast majority of patients with advanced locoregional cervical cancer. The effectiveness of radiation therapy depends on establishing a delicate balance between external beam radiation therapy and brachytherapy, as well as maximizing the distribution of the radiation dose to both malignant and healthy tissue while decreasing the overall treatment duration. Patients treated with radiation therapy alone for stages IIB, IIIB, and IVA had 5-year survival rates of 65–75%, 35–50%, and 5–15%, respectively [27, 28]. This first treatment can increase the efficacy of later intracavitary brachytherapy by lowering the size of the tumor and bringing it back within the dose distribution of brachytherapy. External irradiation is always combined with concomitant chemotherapy to offer a consistent initial dosage to both the primary cervical cancer and any regional spread locations. The objective underlying brachytherapy, a crucial component of definitive radiation therapy, is to follow the inverse square rule in order to provide a higher dose to the cervix and paracervical regions while limiting damage to nearby normal tissue. If you wish to complete radiation therapy in less than 7–8 weeks, avoiding delays between an external beam surgery and an intracavitary procedure is one of the most crucial things to bear in mind [29].

For the majority of patients with an isolated pelvic recurrence after the first therapy with radical hysterectomy alone, definitive radiation is the preferred treatment. Vaginal recurrence is routinely treated with EBRT and brachytherapy, following the same techniques as for patients with vaginal cancer. Recurrences of pelvic wall cancer are frequently treated with EBRT. Certain patients may benefit from surgery combined with intraoperative radiation for local management. A vaginal recurrence is associated with a more favorable prognosis than a pelvic wall recurrence [30]. An isolated central recurrence of the subsequent radiation can be treated surgically in individuals. Due to the difficulty in assessing the extent of pathology following high-dose radiation and the significant risk of major urinary tract complications associated with pelvic surgery, surgical salvage treatment typically requires a pelvic exenteration, most commonly an anterior or complete exenteration [31, 32]. Less invasive procedures, including radical hysterectomy, are reserved for women with cervical cancer or tumors that do not spread into the rectum. In all situations, pelvic exenteration preparation must include a comprehensive medical and radiological evaluation and meticulous counseling of the patient and family regarding the extent of the treatment and postoperative difficulties. PET/CT scans should be performed to rule out the presence of severe pelvic sidewall involvement or extra pelvic metastases. Cancerous infiltration of the pelvic sidewall is a contraindication to exenteration; however, this may be difficult to determine if there is considerable radiation fibrosis.

Patients with unresectable recurrent cervical cancer who have undergone final radiation therapy have few therapeutic options available to them. However, chemotherapy is administered to the majority of patients with unresectable pelvic recurrences following radiation therapy. This results in relatively low response rates and large death rates.

Patients who present symptoms or experience relapses related to sickness in distant organs typically cannot be cured. The treatment for these individuals should focus on reducing their symptoms as much as possible by using effective painkillers and local RT. Tumors can be treated, although the results of treatment are typically very temporary. Metastases can produce pain in various locations, including the bone, brain, lymph nodes, and other areas. Localized RT can successfully treat this discomfort. Individuals who are toward the end of their lives and have an extended disease may find relief from pelvic pain and bleeding by undergoing a course of palliative pelvic radiation [33].

7. Radiation therapy treatment techniques

For external-beam RT, the use of CT-based treatment planning and conformal blocking is considered the standard of care (EBRT). MRI is the best imaging modality for patients with advanced malignancies for evaluating soft tissue and parametrial involvement. PET imaging is effective in individuals who have not been surgically staged to assist in defining the nodal volume of coverage and may be helpful postoperatively to confirm the excision of suspicious nodes.

To reduce treatment setup errors, CT simulation should be performed with the patient in a supine position and a specialized immobilization device. Patients with cancer covering the distal one-half of the vagina (or vaginal primary) should get bilateral inguinal RT, with CT simulation conducted in the "frog-leg" posture to avoid skin fold toxicity. Scans with a slice thickness of ≤3 mm should be acquired. The bladder and rectal filling level seen during simulation should ideally match that found with daily treatments. Consider two scans for the bladder full and empty to create an internal target volume (ITV). Fuse with MRI/PET imaging (if available) to define tumor extent. Treatment with a full bladder can shift the bowel from the treatment field and enhance bowel dosimetry; however, treatment with an empty bladder may be more repeatable and minimizes the absolute fluctuation in bladder volume. To simulate an empty rectum, bowel preparation with an enema might be employed. Because the patient's pelvic vasculature acts as a reference for lymph node placement, intravenous contrast simulation is advised unless medically contraindicated. Implantation of fiducial markers prior to CT simulation or placement of radiopaque markers in the vaginal apex and introitus during simulation are two techniques for increasing target volume identification. Using PO contrast could also help delineate a bowel bag. Consider marking the lower portion of pathology if there is a vaginal extension.

In all settings, effort must be taken to encompass all pelvis regions at risk for pathology. EBRT is delivered using multiple conformal fields or intensity-modulated volumetric techniques, such as IMRT/volumetric-modulated arc therapy (VMAT)/ tomotherapy. Typically, IMRT is used for most post-operative whole pelvis irradiation or extended field RT when inguinal and/or para-aortal nods are treated. Most ongoing clinical trials only utilize IMRT as the standard of EBRT.

For conformal RT, particularly IMRT, the gross target volume (GTV), clinical target volume (CTV), planning target volume (PTV), organs at risk (OARs), internal organ motion, and dose-volume histogram (DVH) have been established. The volume of EBRT should include the gross disease (if present), the parametria, the uterosacral ligaments, a sufficient vaginal margin from the gross disease (at least 3 cm), the presacral lymph nodes, and any additional at-risk nodal volumes. For patients with negative surgical or radiologic imaging of the lymph nodes, the radiation volume should encompass the whole external iliac, internal iliac, obturator, and presacral nodal basins. For individuals thought to be at a greater risk of lymph node involvement (e.g., bulkier tumors; suspected or confirmed lymph nodes localized to the low true pelvis), the radiation dose should be raised to include the common iliacs. In individuals with common iliac and/or para-aortic nodal involvement, pelvic and para-aortic radiation up to the level of the renal vessels is indicated (or even more cephalad as directed by involved nodal distribution). Patients with below one-third vaginal involvement should also have bilateral groins covered. There have been published international consensus guidelines for target volume contouring [34]. The multi-institutional cooperative group phase III NRG-GY006 clinical trial contouring recommendations derived by Nancy lee and colleagues are presented in **Table 5** [35].

For patients with primary cervical cancer who are not candidates for surgery, brachytherapy is a key component of the ultimate treatment plan that they will follow. In this case, either an intracavitary or an interstitial approach will do the trick. GEC-ESTRO recommendations are available for volume-based brachytherapy contouring, and they recommend utilizing CT or MRI to delineate treatment targets [36]. A high-risk MRI-based CTV is defined as the whole cervix in addition to any parametrial or vaginal extension (gray zones). CT-based CTV (high-risk): all central tissue at the level of ring or ovoids, superiorly to internal os, then 1 cm "cone" along tandem above

Target name	Details
GTV	All visible gross disease as assessed by clinical information, physical examination, radiographic studies, endoscopic examination, and biopsy results
CTV 1	GTV + cervix + uterus
CTV 2	Parametria and upper third of the vagina (or upper half if the vagina is clinically involved)
CTV 3	Common, external iliac, internal iliac, and presacral lymph nodes. The upper border should start the aortic bifurcation (approximately L4–L5 interspace). Presacral nodes should be included to the S2–S3 interspace; below this point this nodal volume can be separated into two structures. External iliac nodes should be included to the top of the femoral heads. If there is distal vaginal involvement, the inguinal nodes should be included (from the external iliac nodes to 2 cm caudal to the saphenous/femoral junction). If para-aortic nodes are involved, an extended field should be used, extending the superior border to the L1/L2 interspace or 3 cm cranial to gross disease. CTV3 should be obtained by placing a 7 mm margin around the vessels with inclusion of any adjacent visible lymph nodes, lymphoceles, or surgical clips. This volume should be modified to exclude bone, muscle, and bowel, and should not extend inferior to the ischial tuberosities
CTV-Boost	Gross pelvic lymph nodes. If the patient will receive a parametrial boost, this area should be included
ITV	If an ITV approach is to be used, CTV1 should be delineated on both the full and empty bladder scans and combined to generate the ITV
CTV_4500 or CTV_4760	CTV1 + CTV2 + CTV3 + ITV
PTV1	CTV1 + 15 mm uniform expansion
PTV2	CTV2 + 10 mm uniform expansion
PTV3	CTV3 + 5 mm uniform expansion
PTV4	ITV + 7 mm uniform expansion
PTV_boost	CTV_boost +5 mm uniform expansion
PTV_4500 or PTV_4760	PTV1 + PTV2 + PTV3 + PTV4 + PTV_boost. This should be trimmed up to 3 mm from the skin surface, if necessary, to spare skin. The CTV should be fully encompassed by the PTV

Table 5.
Target delineation for cervical cancer (per NRG-GY006 protocol).

cervix; laterally, include any parametrial extension (gray/white) or clinical vaginal involvement. CT-based CTV (low-risk): all central tissue at the level of ring or ovoids, superiorly to internal os. There are two-point definitions for point-based dosage in brachytherapy: ICRU 38 and 2011 ABS point. Point A is located at the point where the tandem meets the line that connects the peaks of the ovoids or the ring; it is situated 2 cms above and 2 cms to the side of the tandem (point B 5 cm lateral to the tandem). The bladder point is the posterior position of the midfoley balloon after it has been inflated with 7 ml of fluid. The rectal point is located 5 mm posterior to the vaginal wall at the lower intrauterine source. The surface of ovoids or cylinders that make up the vaginal cavity.

In patients with an intact cervix, the original tumor and susceptible regional lymphatics are routinely treated with 45 Gy of definitive EBRT (40–50 Gy). The dose of EBRT would be proportional to the nodal status as assessed by surgery or imaging. The primary cervical tumor is then boosted employing brachytherapy with an additional 30–40 Gy using image guidance (preferred) or to point A (in low dose-rate [LDR] equivalent dose), for a total point A dose of 80 Gy for small-volume cervical tumors or 85 Gy for larger-volume cervical tumors. For highly tiny tumors (clinically inoperable IA1 or IA2), 75–80 Gy EQD2 D90 dosages may be explored. Grossly affected, unresected lymph nodes may be boosted with an additional 10–15 Gy of highly conformal EBRT. When employing imaging guidance for EBRT, care must be made to exclude or severely restrict the amount of normal tissue inside the high-dose zones (**Tables 6–8**).

The presence of one or more pathologic risk factors following a prior hysterectomy may justify the use of adjuvant RT. The following should be covered at a minimum: the top 3–4 cms of the vaginal cuff, the parametria, and surrounding nodal regions (such as the external and internal iliac, obturator, and presacral nodes). The radiation field's superior edge should be increased accordingly for confirmed nodal metastases. In general, 45–50 Gy in conventional fractionation is advised for IMRT. Four grossly

Source	External beam organ	Type	Volume/dose
QUANTEC	Bowel bag	Vol (mL)	≤195 cc above 45 Gy
Institutional Series	Duodenum	Vol (mL)	<5–15 cc above 55 Gy
RTOG	Femoral heads	Vol (%)	<15% above 30 Gy; <50% above 30 Gy
GEC-ESTRO	Femoral heads	Dose max	50 Gy

Table 6.
GYN tissue tolerances.

Source	External beam organ	Type	Volume/dose
TIME-C	Bowel bag	Vol (%)	Goal <30% above 40 Gy
TIME-C	Bladder	Vol (%)	Goal <35% above 45 Gy
TIME-C	Bone marrow	Vol (%)	Goal <90% receives 10 Gy
TIME-C	Bone marrow	Vol (%)	Goal <37% receives 40 Gy
TIME-C	Rectum	Vol (%)	Goal <80% above 40 Gy

Table 7.
Post-hysterectomy dose constraints.

Source	Organ	Type	Volume/dose
GEC-ESTRO	Rectum	Vol (mL)	<2 cc above 65 Gy total $EQD2_3$ (limit 75 Gy)
GEC-ESTRO	Sigmoid	Vol (mL)	<2 cc above 70 Gy total $EQD2_3$ (limit 75 Gy)
GEC-ESTRO	Bladder	Vol (mL)	<2 cc above 80 Gy total $EQD2_3$ (limit 90 Gy)
GEC-ESTRO	Bowel	Vol (mL)	<2 cc above 70 Gy total $EQD2_3$ (limit 75 Gy)
GEC-ESTRO	Recto-vaginal point	Vol (mL)	<2 cc above 65 Gy total $EQD2_3$ (limit 75 Gy)
GECESTRO (vaginal cancer)	Vaginal surface	Dose max	<130 Gy total $EQD2_3$ (limit 140 Gy)

Table 8.
Brachytherapy for cervical cancer dose constraints.

affected, unresected lymph nodes may be considered for boosting with an extra 10–20 Gy of highly conformal EBRT.

In exceptional cases, patients whose anatomy or tumor geometry makes intracavitary brachytherapy impossible may be effectively treated with an interstitial approach; however, such interstitial brachytherapy should be accomplished only by individuals and institutions with the required knowledge and training, and early referral for prompt use of own knowledge and experience is essential. In certain post-hysterectomy patients (particularly those with positive or near vaginal mucosal surgical margins), vaginal cylinder brachytherapy may be utilized as an adjunct to external beam radiation treatment (EBRT). Typically, the prescription is applied to the vaginal surface or 5 mm below it. Typical fractionation strategies include 5.5 Gy 2 fractions at 5 mm or 6 Gy 3 fractions at the vaginal surface.

SBRT is the most certain technique among all EBRT modalities in terms of its ability to simulate a brachytherapy dose distribution with a steep dose gradient and, as a result, achieve the same treatment outcomes as ICB, at least theoretically. Although being under investigation and recommended by few retrospective reviews, SBRT is not regarded as a reasonable alternative to brachytherapy for routine use.

8. Post-radiation toxicity and complications

In the scientific literature, the terms “acute toxicity” and “late toxicity” are defined in a variety of ways. In certain contexts, the term “acute toxicity” refers to the development of unfavorable consequences that take place both during the course of treatment and up to 42, 60, or 90 days following the completion of radiation therapy. Late toxicity is when an impact does not show up for 90 days or even years after it has been exposed to something. Although complications are reported to be slightly higher (10–15%) in patients with the locally progressed disease, the incidence of late sequelae in individuals with early-stage cervical cancer treated with RT is approximately 3.5%. However, complications are reported to be slightly higher in patients with more advanced diseases. The logic for this variance is straightforward: as the clinical stage of a patient continues to advance, the total dosage to central structures has a tendency to increase (e.g., 85–90 Gy are administered to the cervix in clinical stage III and IV patients). We can conclude that the risk of problems is related to the clinical stage, the volume of tissue being treated, the patient's anatomy, and the total dosage supplied to certain tissues [37].

Mild tiredness and mild to moderate diarrhea are common side effects of pelvic radiation but may be managed with antidiarrheal drugs. Some patients may also have mild bladder discomfort, which can be a sign of a urinary tract infection. Patients receiving treatment with extended fields may experience nausea, stomach discomfort, and a reduction in peripheral blood cell counts. Concurrent chemotherapy considerably increases the risk of hematologic and gastrointestinal problems. The most prevalent sexual problems after irradiation are ovarian insufficiency in premenopausal women and vaginal stenosis in vaginal radiation patients. Vaginal stenosis is a tightening or narrowing of the vaginal canal that can interfere with a physical exam or sexual function. Its prevalence ranges from 20 to 88% [38]. Ovarian failure occurs in all premenopausal individuals treated with pelvic radiation unless the ovaries have been transferred. Uterine perforation, fever, and the common complications associated with anesthesia are all possible side effects of intracavitary brachytherapy. Thromboembolic events are uncommon.

Estimates of the risk of late sequelae from radical radiation vary depending on the grading system, length of follow-up, calculation method, treatment approach, and prevalence of risk variables in the study group. Complication rates in individuals with extremely locally advanced pathologies may be greater due in part to tissue loss induced by infiltrative malignancy. Rectal complications are most frequent in the first 3 years after therapy and include bleeding, stricture, ulceration, and fistula. Small intestinal obstruction is a rare consequence of conventional radiation in patients with no additional risk factors. Patients with open transperitoneal lymph node dissection have a considerably higher risk of small intestinal blockage. A history of pelvic inflammatory disease or peritonitis, thin body habitus, heavy smoking, and the use of high doses or large volumes for external-beam irradiation, particularly with low-energy treatment beams and large daily fraction sizes, can all increase the risk of small bowel complications in patients treated for cervical cancer [37].

High doses of radiation can produce persistent myelosuppressive effects and a lower tolerance to the effects of chemotherapy. These effects are caused when the microenvironment of the bone marrow is altered. Prospective analyses indicated a 25% prevalence of hematological damage >G3 when cisplatin-based chemoradiotherapy was utilized. Irradiating an expanded field that encompasses the para-aortic lymph node covering leads to greater irradiation of total bone marrow and, as a result, a higher incidence of hematological damage. This outcome must be examined and managed since it predisposes patients to infections, repeated hospitalizations, multiple transfusions, and delays in obtaining therapy [39, 40]. Loren K Mell reported about bone marrow-sparing IMRT in 2008. The report concluded that BMS-IMRT reduced the irradiation of pelvic bone marrow compared with the four-field box technique [41]. In order to find the most effective method to lessen the hematological toxicity associated with concurrent chemoradiotherapy (cCRT) for cervical cancer, De-Yang Yu and his colleagues set out to investigate the dosimetric characteristics of a variety of bone marrow-sparing strategies and radiation technologies in 2020. Their ultimate goal was to identify the most effective method. The scientists came to the conclusion that the IMRT plan that achieved the best sparing while still giving enough coverage of the target volume was the one that excluded the bone marrow from the radiation treatment and treated the pelvic bones with discrete dose-volume limitations. In addition, among all of the more recent radiation treatment systems, the VMAT has shown itself to be the most successful in terms of preserving bone marrow while still providing overall efficacy. Patients with cervical cancer might benefit from this treatment technique since it can potentially lessen the hematological toxicity they experience. By using this method, we are able to increase the effectiveness of radiation and reduce the need for expensive functional imaging of active bone marrow [42].

9. Ongoing clinical trials and future perspectives

On October 2021, the highly anticipated KEYNOTE-826 trial confirmed that there was a survival benefit of adding immunotherapy in the form of a drug called Pembrolizumab to chemotherapy for patients with persistent, recurrent, or metastatic cancer. The KEYNOTE-A18 trial is an ENGOT (European Network for Gynecological Oncological Trial groups) and GOG partners collaboration. It is a randomized phase 3 trial with chemoradiotherapy with or without pembrolizumab for high-risk locally advanced cervical cancer. And 980 patients are anticipated to receive pembrolizumab on day 1 of a 3-week cycle for 5 cycles, followed by pembrolizumab on day 1 of a 6-week cycle for 15 cycles. The primary outcome is progression-free survival (PFS) and overall survival (OS) [43]. Dr. Tewari is researching high-risk individuals, patients with stage IIIB or IIIC positive lymph nodes, or even aortic nodes, and has randomized them to chemotherapy, radiation, placebo versus durvalumab, added both in the radiation phase and the maintenance phase for up to 24 months. This study is known as CALLA, and it is enrolled. There are 714 subjects listed on clinicaltrials.g ov, and the trial has been closed since December 2020 [44].

In addition, the currently approved therapies for cervical cancer are accompanied by debilitating side effects and tumor drug resistance. This is the case despite significant breakthroughs in the utilization of combination medicines. To increase the efficacy of single-agent therapies for cervical cancer, there is a pressing need to discover new and better medications. Immunotherapy, targeted therapy, and genetic methods such as CRISPR/Cas9 and RNAi are among the various cervical cancer therapies now under investigation. These are only a few instances of the treatment options available. Chemotherapy and radiation therapy are other treatment choices to explore. The majority of these therapies are still in the research phase, and the alternatives they provide are more costly. Identification of non-cancer medicines that target host factors that, in conjunction with HPV oncoproteins, notably E6 and E7, promote cervical cancer progression is one method that may lead to timely medication development at an acceptable and cheap price. This strategy, which combines a targeted approach with medication redirection, is appealing because it should find pharmaceuticals with far fewer adverse effects than conventional cancer therapies. This makes the idea more appealing. Due to the extensive study of their safety profiles, it is anticipated that they will enter clinical trials quickly [45].

Acknowledgements

I want to thank the people working at EVEX hospitals-Krystyna Kiel Oncology Center for their encouragement and advice that led to the completion of this paper.

I also thank my friends for their encouragement and words of advice. Special thanks to my mentor—Krystyna Kiel. Finally, if not for my family, who supports me all the time, I would never be able to work on this extraordinary project.

Conflict of interest

The author declared no potential conflicts of interest with respect to the research, authorship, and/or publication of this article. This research did not receive a specific grant from funding agencies in the public, commercial, or not-for-profit sectors.

Author details

Eter Natelauri
EVEX Hospitals-Krystyna Kiel Oncology Center, Kutaisi, Georgia

*Address all correspondence to: enatelauri@yahoo.com

References

[1] Cervical Cancer. Www.who.int. Retrieved December 1, 2022. Available from: www.who.int/health-topics/cervical-cancer#tab=tab_1

[2] SEER. Cancer of the Cervix Uteri—Cancer Stat Facts. Available from: seer.cancer.gov/statfacts/html/cervix.html [Accessed: November 25, 2022]

[3] Agency for Research on Cancer (IARC), The International Global Cancer Observatory. Global Cancer Observatory. Available from: gco.iarc.fr [Accessed: November 25, 2022]

[4] Cannistra SA, Niloff JM. Cancer of the uterine cervix. The New England Journal of Medicine. 1996;**334**(16):1030-1038. DOI: 10.1056/NEJM199604183341606

[5] Thomas DB, Ray RM. Oral contraceptives and invasive adenocarcinomas and adenosquamous carcinomas of the uterine cervix. The World Health Organization Collaborative Study of Neoplasia and Steroid Contraceptives. American Journal of Epidemiology. 1996;**144**(3): 281-289. DOI: 10.1093/oxfordjournals.aje.a008923

[6] Strayer David S, Rubin's pathology: Clinicopathologic foundations of medicine. Jefferson Faculty Books. 2015. Available from: https://jdc.jefferson.edu/jeffersonfacultybooks/66

[7] Solomon D, Davey D, Kurman R, Moriarty A, O'Connor D, Prey M, et al. The 2001 Bethesda system: Terminology for reporting results of cervical cytology. JAMA. 2002;**287**(16):2114-2119. DOI: 10.1001/jama.287.16.2114

[8] Katki HA, Schiffman M, Castle PE, Fetterman B, Poitras NE, Lorey T, et al. Five-year risks of CIN 3+ and cervical cancer among women with HPV-positive and HPV-negative high-grade Pap results. Journal of Lower Genital Tract Disease. 2013;**17**(5 Suppl 1):S50-S55. DOI: 10.1097/LGT.0b013e3182854282

[9] Katki HA, Schiffman M, Castle PE, Fetterman B, Poitras NE, Lorey T, et al. Five-year risks of CIN 3+ and cervical cancer among women with HPV testing of ASC-US Pap results. Journal of Lower Genital Tract Disease. 2013;**17**(5 Suppl 1):S36-S42. DOI: 10.1097/LGT.0b013e3182854253

[10] Nayar R, Wilbur DC. The Bethesda System for reporting cervical cytology: A historical perspective. Acta Cytologica. 2017;**61**(4–5):359-372. DOI: 10.1159/000477556

[11] Robert ME, Fu YS. Squamous cell carcinoma of the uterine cervix–a review with emphasis on prognostic factors and unusual variants. Seminars in Diagnostic Pathology. 1990;**7**(3):173-189

[12] Peters RK, Chao A, Mack TM, Thomas D, Bernstein L, Henderson BE. Increased frequency of adenocarcinoma of the uterine cervix in young women in Los Angeles County. Journal of the National Cancer Institute. 1986;**76**(3): 423-428

[13] Plentl AA, Friedman EA. Lymphatic system of the female genitalia. The morphologic basis of oncologic diagnosis and therapy. Major Problems in Obstetrics and Gynecology. 1971;**2**:1-223

[14] Kraima AC, Derks M, Smit NN, Van Munsteren JC, Van der Velden J, Kenter GG, et al. Lymphatic drainage pathways from the cervix uteri: Implications for radical hysterectomy? Gynecologic

Oncology. 2014;**132**(1):107-113. DOI: 10.1016/j.ygyno.2013.10.030

[15] Salvo G, Ramirez PT, Levenback CF, Munsell MF, Euscher ED, Soliman PT, et al. Sensitivity and negative predictive value for sentinel lymph node biopsy in women with early-stage cervical cancer. Gynecologic Oncology. 2017;**145**(1):96-101. DOI: 10.1016/j.ygyno.2017.02.005

[16] Fagundes H, Perez CA, Grigsby PW, Lockett MA. Distant metastases after irradiation alone in carcinoma of the uterine cervix. International Journal of Radiation Oncology, Biology, Physics. 1992;**24**(2):197-204. DOI: 10.1016/0360-3016(92)90671-4

[17] Kim RY, Weppelmann B, Salter MM, Brascho DJ. Skeletal metastases from cancer of the uterine cervix: Frequency, patterns, and radiotherapeutic significance. International Journal of Radiation Oncology, Biology, Physics. 1987;**13**(5):705-708. DOI: 10.1016/0360-3016(87)90288-4

[18] Bhatla N, Aoki D, Sharma DN, Sankaranarayanan R. Cancer of the cervix uteri: 2021 update. International Journal of Gynaecology and Obstetrics: The Official Organ of the International Federation of Gynaecology and Obstetrics. 2021;**155**((Suppl 1)):28-44. DOI: 10.1002/ijgo.13865

[19] Viswanathan AN, Dizon DS, Gien LT, Koh WJ. Cervical cancer. In: Leonard L. Gunderson, Joel E. Tepper, editors. Clinical Radiation Oncology (Fourth Edition). Elsevier; 2015. 4pp. 1173-1202.e6. DOI: 10.1016/B978-0-323-24098-7.00058-7. ISBN: 9780323240987. Available from: https://www.sciencedirect.com/science/article/pii/B9780323240987000587

[20] Creasman WT, Zaino RJ, Major FJ, DiSaia PJ, Hatch KD, Homesley HD. Early invasive carcinoma of the cervix (3 to 5 mm invasion): Risk factors and prognosis. A Gynecologic Oncology Group study. American Journal of Obstetrics and Gynecology. 1998;**178**(Pt 1):62-65. DOI: 10.1016/s0002-9378(98)70628-3

[21] Pareja R, Rendón GJ, Sanz-Lomana CM, Monzón O, Ramirez PT. Surgical, oncological, and obstetrical outcomes after abdominal radical trachelectomy—A systematic literature review. Gynecologic Oncology. 2013;**131**(1):77-82. DOI: 10.1016/j.ygyno.2013.06.010

[22] Grigsby PW, Perez CA. Radiotherapy alone for medically inoperable carcinoma of the cervix: Stage IA and carcinoma in situ. International Journal of Radiation Oncology, Biology, Physics. 1991;**21**(2):375-378. DOI: 10.1016/0360-3016(91)90785-3

[23] Rotman M, Sedlis A, Piedmonte MR, Bundy B, Lentz SS, Muderspach LI, et al. A phase III randomized trial of postoperative pelvic irradiation in stage IB cervical carcinoma with poor prognostic features: Follow-up of a gynecologic oncology group study. International Journal of Radiation Oncology, Biology, Physics. 2006;**65**(1):169-176. DOI: 10.1016/j.ijrobp.2005.10.019

[24] Alvarez RD, Gelder MS, Gore H, Soong SJ, Partridge EE. Radical hysterectomy in the treatment of patients with bulky early stage carcinoma of the cervix uteri. Surgery, Gynecology & Obstetrics. 1993;**176**(6):539-542

[25] Bloss JD, Berman ML, Mukhererjee J, Manetta A, Emma D, Ramsanghani NS, et al. Bulky stage IB cervical carcinoma managed by primary radical hysterectomy followed by tailored radiotherapy. Gynecologic Oncology.

1992;**47**(1):21-27. DOI: 10.1016/0090-8258(92)90069-u

[26] Landoni F, Maneo A, Colombo A, Placa F, Milani R, Perego P, et al. Randomised study of radical surgery versus radiotherapy for stage Ib-IIa cervical cancer. Lancet (London, England). 1997;**350**(9077):535-540. DOI: 10.1016/S0140-6736(97)02250-2

[27] Logsdon MD, Eifel PJ. FIGO IIIB squamous cell carcinoma of the cervix: An analysis of prognostic factors emphasizing the balance between external beam and intracavitary radiation therapy. International Journal of Radiation Oncology, Biology, Physics. 1999;**43**(4):763-775. DOI: 10.1016/s0360-3016(98)00482-9

[28] Eifel PJ, Morris M, Wharton JT, Oswald MJ. The influence of tumor size and morphology on the outcome of patients with FIGO stage IB squamous cell carcinoma of the uterine cervix. International Journal of Radiation Oncology, Biology, Physics. 1994;**29**(1):9-16. DOI: 10.1016/0360-3016(94)90220-8

[29] Fyles A, Keane TJ, Barton M, Simm J. The effect of treatment duration in the local control of cervix cancer. Radiotherapy and Oncology: Journal of the European Society for Therapeutic Radiology and Oncology. 1992;**25**(4):273-279. DOI: 10.1016/0167-8140(92)90247-r

[30] Mahé MA, Gérard JP, Dubois JB, Roussel A, Bussières E, Delannes M, et al. Intraoperative radiation therapy in recurrent carcinoma of the uterine cervix: Report of the French intraoperative group on 70 patients. International Journal of Radiation Oncology, Biology, Physics. 1996;**34**(1):21-26. DOI: 10.1016/0360-3016(95)02089-6

[31] Maneo A, Landoni F, Cormio G, Colombo A, Mangioni C. Radical hysterectomy for recurrent or persistent cervical cancer following radiation therapy. International Journal of Gynecological Cancer: Official Journal of the International Gynecological Cancer Society. 1999;**9**(4):295-301. DOI: 10.1046/j.1525-1438.1999.99037.x

[32] Coleman RL, Keeney ED, Freedman RS, Burke TW, Eifel PJ, Rutledge FN. Radical hysterectomy for recurrent carcinoma of the uterine cervix after radiotherapy. Gynecologic Oncology. 1994;**55**(1):29-35. DOI: 10.1006/gyno.1994.1242

[33] Natelauri E, Kiel K, Natelauri T, Liluashvili T, Badzgaradze T, Batsikadze J, et al. Palliative split-course pelvic radiotherapy for symptomatic cervical cancer. Medical Science and Discovery. 2022;**9**(4):214-219. DOI: 10.36472/msd.v9i4.704

[34] Lim K, Small W Jr, Portelance L, Creutzberg C, Jürgenliemk-Schulz IM, Mundt A, et al. Consensus guidelines for delineation of clinical target volume for intensity-modulated pelvic radiotherapy for the definitive treatment of cervix cancer. International Journal of Radiation Oncology, Biology, Physics. 2011;**79**(2):348-355. DOI: 10.1016/j.ijrobp.2009.10.075

[35] Testing the Addition of a New Anti-Cancer Drug, Triapine, to the Usual Chemotherapy Treatment (Cisplatin) During Radiation Therapy for Advanced-Stage Cervical and Vaginal Cancers. Available from: https://clinicaltrials.gov/ct2/show/NCT02466971

[36] Pötter R, Haie-Meder C, Van Limbergen E, Barillot I, De Brabandere M, Dimopoulos J, et al. Recommendations from gynaecological

(GYN) GEC ESTRO working group (II): Concepts and terms in 3D image-based treatment planning in cervix cancer brachytherapy-3D dose volume parameters and aspects of 3D image-based anatomy, radiation physics, radiobiology. Radiotherapy and Oncology: Journal of the European Society for Therapeutic Radiology and Oncology. 2006;**78**(1):67-77. DOI: 10.1016/j.radonc.2005.11.014

[37] Eifel PJ, Jhingran A, Bodurka DC, Levenback C, Thames H. Correlation of smoking history and other patient characteristics with major complications of pelvic radiation therapy for cervical cancer. Journal of Clinical Oncology : Official Journal of the American Society of Clinical Oncology. 2002;**20**(17): 3651-3657. DOI: 10.1200/ JCO.2002.10.128

[38] Keys HM, Bundy BN, Stehman FB, Muderspach LI, Chafe WE, Suggs CL 3rd, et al. Cisplatin, radiation, and adjuvant hysterectomy compared with radiation and adjuvant hysterectomy for bulky stage IB cervical carcinoma. The New England Journal of Medicine. 1999; **340**(15):1154-1161. DOI: 10.1056/ NEJM199904153401503

[39] Mauch P, Constine L, Greenberger J, Knospe W, Sullivan J, Liesveld JL, et al. Hematopoietic stem cell compartment: Acute and late effects of radiation therapy and chemotherapy. International Journal of Radiation Oncology, Biology, Physics. 1995;**31**(5):1319-1339. DOI: 10.1016/0360-3016(94)00430-S

[40] Small W Jr, Winter K, Levenback C, Iyer R, Gaffney D, Asbell S, et al. Extended-field irradiation and intracavitary brachytherapy combined with cisplatin chemotherapy for cervical cancer with positive para-aortic or high common iliac lymph nodes: Results of ARM 1 of RTOG 0116. International Journal of Radiation Oncology, Biology, Physics. 2007;**68**(4):1081-1087. DOI: 10.1016/j.ijrobp.2007.01.026

[41] Mell LK, Tiryaki H, Ahn KH, Mundt AJ, Roeske JC, Aydogan B. Dosimetric comparison of bone marrow-sparing intensity-modulated radiotherapy versus conventional techniques for treatment of cervical cancer. International Journal of Radiation Oncology, Biology, Physics. 2008;**71**(5):1504-1510. DOI: 10.1016/ j.ijrobp.2008.04.046

[42] Yu DY, Bai YL, Feng Y, Wang L, Yun WK, Li X, et al. Which bone marrow sparing strategy and radiotherapy technology is most beneficial in bone marrow-sparing intensity modulated radiation therapy for patients with cervical cancer? Frontiers in Oncology. 2020;**10**:554241. DOI: 10.3389/fonc.2020.554241

[43] Efficacy and safety study of first-line treatment with pembrolizumab (MK-3475) plus chemotherapy versus placebo plus chemotherapy in women with persistent, recurrent, or metastatic cervical cancer. ClinicalTrials.gov. n.d.. Available from: https://clinicaltrials.gov/ ct2/show/NCT03635567

[44] Study of durvalumab with chemoradiotherapy for women with locally advanced cervical cancer (Calla). ClinicalTrials.gov. n.d. Available from: https://clinicaltrials.gov/ct2/show/ NCT03830866

[45] Burmeister CA, Khan SF, Schäfer G, Mbatani N, Adams T, Moodley J, et al. Cervical cancer therapies: Current challenges and future perspectives. Tumour Virus Research. 2022;**13**:200238. DOI: 10.1016/j.tvr.2022.200238

Chapter 5

Evaluation of Patients for Radiotherapy for Prostate Adenocarcinoma

Jonathan B. Wallach, Chana Stern, Michael Karp and David L. Schwartz

Abstract

Prostate adenocarcinoma is the most common non-cutaneous malignancy among men in the United States, and the second leading cause of death. However, most prostate adenocarcinoma diagnoses are now diagnosed at early stages and are curable, or if they recur, are associated with such long survival times that the patients usually succumb to competing co-morbidities. This chapter would discuss a brief history of prostate cancer evaluation and its pertinence today, including the Gleason scoring system, advent of PSA testing, and development of the NCCN classification system that is used today. Alternative classification systems, such as the UCSF-CAPRA scoring system, would also be discussed. The latter half of the chapter will discuss the evolution from personalized medicine to precision medicine, including PSMA imaging and prostate cancer genomics, with ongoing trials and future directions. Furthermore, included within this chapter would be a discussion of selecting appropriate men for active surveillance, and appropriate regimens for active surveillance.

Keywords: epidemiology, clinicopathologic risk factors, risk stratification, genomics, prostate adenocarcinoma

1. Introduction

Prostate adenocarcinoma is the second most common diagnosed malignancy and the fifth leading cause of cancer death among men worldwide in 2020, with an estimated 1,414,259 new cases reported in men, along with 375,000 deaths [1]. The incidence and mortality rate of prostate cancer correlates with increasing age, with the average age at diagnosis being 66 years old [2]. The highest incidences of prostate cancer were in North America, Southern Africa, Northern and Western Europe, the Caribbean, and Australia/New Zealand; the lowest incidence rates were in Asia and North Africa.

In the United States between 2012 and 2017, the incidence rate of prostate cancer for all races combined was 104/100,000 persons; it was 97/100,000 for non-Hispanic whites, 173/100,000 for blacks, and 52/100,000 for Asian/Pacific Islanders. The mortality rate for all races combined was 19/100,000 persons; 18/100,000 for non-Hispanic whites, 38/100,000 for blacks, and 18/100,000 for Asian/Pacific Islanders.

2. PSA testing

In the United States, the incidence of prostate cancer increased in the early 1990s due to the widespread use of prostate-specific antigen (PSA) monitoring that was formally approved by the Food & Drug Administration in 1986, and dramatically increased the detection of asymptomatic/early-stage disease. Incidence rates declined suddenly between 2007 and 2014, and stabilized around 2016. In 2012, the United States Preventive Services Task Force (USPSTF) recommended against routine PSA screening for prostate cancer due to overdiagnosis and overtreatment that could potentially affect quality of life for patients. This recommendation likely led to the decrease in the overall reported incidence rates, but later resulted in an increase in the incidence of advanced-stage disease [3]. In 2018, the USPSTF released updated guidelines for PSA screening as follows: [4].

1. For men between the ages of 55–69, the decision to be screened should be on an individualized basis, and patients are encouraged to discuss the potential risks and benefits of screening with their physicians including overdiagnosis and overtreatment, which can lead to long-term complications.

2. Men 70 years or older are recommended to not undergo PSA screening.

However, the American Cancer Society has released guidelines that are more in favor of PSA testing, recommending that the decision for PSA testing should take place as follows: [5].

1. Age 50 for men who are at average risk of prostate cancer and are expected to live at least 10 more years

2. Age 45 for men at high risk of developing prostate cancer. This includes African Americans and men who have a first-degree relative (father or brother) diagnosed with prostate cancer at an early age (younger than 65).

3. Age 40 for men at even higher risk (those with more than one first-degree relative who had prostate cancer at an early age).

3. Development of the Gleason score

The Gleason grading system for prostate adenocarcinoma originated in the 1960s from a randomized prospective study performed at the Veterans Administration that included nearly 3000 patients. Dr. Donald Gleason detailed and summarized the histological growth patterns (grades) of prostate adenocarcinoma, and the correlation with clinical data such as staging and prognosis were analyzed.

At the 2014 International Society of Urological Pathology Consensus Conference, a new prostate adenocarcinoma grading system was developed from the latest Gleason scoring system that was last revised in 2005, which included a new system of Grade Groups from Gleason scores 1–5, as follows: [6].

Grade Group 1: Gleason score ≤ 6; only individual discrete well-formed glands.

Grade Group 2: Gleason score $3 + 4 = 7$; predominantly well-formed glands with lesser components of poorly formed/fused/cribriform glands.

Grade Group 3: Gleason score 4 + 3 = 7; predominantly poorly formed/fused/cribriform glands with lesser component of well-formed glands

- For cases with >95% poorly formed/fused/cribriform glands or lack of glands on a core or at radical prostatectomy, the component of <5% well-formed glands is not factored into the grade.

Grade Group 4: Gleason score 4 + 4 = 8, 3 + 5 = 8, 5 + 3 = 8

- Only poorly-formed/fused/cribriform glands; or
- Predominantly well-formed glands and lesser component lacking glands (poorly formed/fused/cribriform glands can be a more minor component); or
- Predominantly lacking glands and lesser component of well-formed glands (poorly formed/fused/cribriform glands can be a more minor component)

Grade Group 5: Gleason score 9–10; lack gland formation (or with necrosis) with or without poorly formed/fused/cribriform glands.

4. Assessment of prostate cancer risk

4.1 D'Amico risk classification of prostate cancer

In 1998, Dr. Anthony D'Amico created a model that stratified patients with prostate cancer into those with a low, intermediate, or high risk of biochemical recurrence-free survival after surgery based on Gleason score at biopsy, clinical tumor-nodal-metastasis (TNM) stage, and pre-operative PSA level, as follows, in **Table 1** [7].

4.2 Modern NCCN classification system

The modern National Comprehensive Cancer Network (NCCN) classification system includes a six-tier system, with very low-risk, low-risk, favorable intermediate-risk (FIR), unfavorable intermediate-risk (UIR), high-risk, and very high-risk (see **Figure 1**) [8].

Importantly, this new system divides the heterogenous group of intermediate-risk prostate adenocarcinoma into favorable and unfavorable classifications. This bifurcation is based on research led by Drs. Zachary Zumsteg and Michael Zelefsky at Memorial Sloan Kettering Cancer Center between 1992 and 2007, on 1208 patients with intermediate-risk prostate cancer treated with dose-escalated external beam radiotherapy (EBRT) to 81 Gy or 86.4 Gy in 1.8 Gy daily fractions with or without

Low-Risk	Intermediate-Risk	High-Risk
Gleason Score ≤ 6, and PSA <10 ng/ml, and Clinical Stage ≤T2a	Gleason Score of 7, or PSA of 10 to <20 ng/ml, or Clinical Stage T2b	Gleason Score ≥ 8, or PSA ≥20 ng/ml, or Clinical Stage ≥T2c

Table 1.
Original D'Amico three-tier classification system.

National Comprehensive Cancer Network® NCCN

NCCN Guidelines Version 1.2023
Prostate Cancer

NCCN Guidelines Index
Table of Contents
Discussion

INITIAL RISK STRATIFICATION AND STAGING WORKUP FOR CLINICALLY LOCALIZED DISEASE[e]

Risk Group	Clinical/Pathologic Features See Staging (ST-1)	Additional Evaluation[h,i]	Initial Therapy
Very low[f]	Has all of the following: • cT1c • Grade Group 1 • PSA <10 ng/mL • Fewer than 3 prostate biopsy fragments/cores positive, ≤50% cancer in each fragment/core[g] • PSA density <0.15 ng/mL/g	• Confirmatory testing can be used to assess the appropriateness of active surveillance (See PROS-F 2 of 5)	See PROS-3
Low[f]	Has all of the following but does not qualify for very low risk: • cT1–cT2a • Grade Group 1 • PSA <10 ng/mL	• Confirmatory testing can be used to assess the appropriateness of active surveillance (See PROS-F 2 of 5)	See PROS-4
Intermediate[f]	Has all of the following: • No high-risk group features • No very-high-risk group features • Has one or more intermediate risk factors (IRFs): ▸ cT2b–cT2c ▸ Grade Group 2 or 3 ▸ PSA 10–20 ng/mL Favorable intermediate: Has all of the following: • 1 IRF • Grade Group 1 or 2 • <50% biopsy cores positive (eg, <6 of 12 cores)[g]	• Confirmatory testing can be used to assess the appropriateness of active surveillance (See PROS-F 2 of 5)	See PROS-5
	Unfavorable intermediate: Has one or more of the following: • 2 or 3 IRFs • Grade Group 3 • ≥ 50% biopsy cores positive (eg, ≥ 6 of 12 cores)[g]	Bone and soft tissue imaging[j,k] • If regional or distant metastases are found, see PROS-8 or PROS-12	See PROS-6
High	Has no very-high-risk features and has exactly one high-risk feature: • cT3a OR • Grade Group 4 or Grade Group 5 OR • PSA >20 ng/mL	Bone and soft tissue imaging[j,k] • If regional or distant metastases are found, see PROS-8 or PROS-12	See PROS-7
Very high	Has at least one of the following: • cT3b–cT4 • Primary Gleason pattern 5 • 2 or 3 high-risk features • >4 cores with Grade Group 4 or 5	Bone and soft tissue imaging[j,k] • If regional or distant metastases are found, see PROS-8 or PROS-12	See PROS-7

Figure 1.
NCCN prostate initial risk stratification and staging work-up for clinically localized disease [8].

short-term androgen deprivation therapy (ADT) [9]. FIR prostate cancer was defined as having NCCN intermediate-risk disease and all the following: a single intermediate risk factor, Gleason 3 + 4 = 7, and < 50% of biopsy cores positive. UIR prostate cancer was classified as any intermediate-risk patient with at least one of the following: primary Gleason pattern of 4, ≥50% of biopsy cores positive, PSA ≥10, and cT2b-cT2c. The results demonstrated that patients with UIR disease had a 2.4x increase in PSA recurrence, 4.3x increase in distant metastases, and 7.4x increases in prostate cancer-specific mortality; therefore, it was concluded that a bifurcation could be made within the intermediate-risk category.

4.3 UCSF-CAPRA scoring system

The UCSF-Cancer of the Prostate Risk Assessment (CAPRA) score is another model developed to predict the aggressiveness of a diagnosed prostate adenocarcinoma, including primary endpoints such as prostate cancer–specific mortality, all-cause mortality, and metastatic disease in patients post-treatment (see **Figure 2** and **Table 2**) [10].

5. Estimates of life expectancy

Upon consultation, an estimation of life expectancy is crucial for shared decision-making between a physician and patient, as prostate cancer can often be an indolent disease prone to overtreatment, leading to unnecessary side effects. Various nomograms are available to assist in estimating life expectancy, and aiding these decisions prior to treatment. For example, the Memorial Sloan Kettering Cancer Center website has a "Male Life Expectancy" calculator [11]. Nevertheless, this estimation should be

Actuarial survival outcomes stratified by Cancer of the Prostate Risk Assessment (CAPRA) score*

	Metastasis-free interval, % likelihood (95% CI)		Prostate cancer-specific survival, % likelihood (95% CI)		Overall survival, % likelihood (95% CI)	
CAPRA score(s)	5 y	10 y	5 y	10 y	5 y	10 y
0	100	100	100	100	100	100
1	99.5 (98.8 to 99.8)	99.0 (97.1 to 99.6)	99.7 (99.3 to 99.9)	98.2 (93.3 to 99.5)	93.0 (91.2 to 94.5)	76.7 (69.7 to 82.4)
2	99.1 (98.5 to 99.5)	96.9 (94.7 to 98.2)	99.8 (99.3 to 99.9)	96.7 (94.2 to 98.1)	92.1 (90.7 to 93.4)	69.1 (64.9 to 73.0)
3	97.3 (96.3 to 98.1)	95.5 (93.7 to 96.8)	99.1 (98.3 to 99.5)	94.4 (91.7 to 96.3)	90.2 (88.4 to 91.7)	64.1 (59.8 to 68.0)
4	97.2 (95.8 to 98.2)	92.7 (89.2 to 95.1)	98.4 (97.2 to 99.1)	89.7 (84.9 to 93.0)	91.0 (88.7 to 92.8)	57.9 (52.1 to 63.3)
5	95.4 (93.2 to 96.9)	88.7 (83.3 to 92.4)	97.8 (95.9 to 98.8)	87.4 (81.1 to 91.7)	89.3 (86.3 to 91.6)	52.1 (45.2 to 58.5)
6	93.6 (90.9 to 95.6)	84.7 (78.4 to 89.3)	95.3 (92.6 to 97.0)	79.3 (71.8 to 85.0)	83.2 (79.2 to 86.5)	45.7 (38.7 to 52.4)
7	91.1 (87.3 to 93.8)	84.6 (76.7 to 90.0)	94.1 (90.3 to 96.5)	78.6 (67.9 to 86.1)	77.0 (71.4 to 81.6)	36.3 (28.0 to 44.7)
8–10	83.0 (77.9 to 87.1)	79.2 (72.8 to 84.3)	88.7 (83.6 to 92.4)	78.9 (70.0 to 85.4)	72.4 (66.0 to 77.8)	41.5 (33.1 to 49.8)
0–2	99.3 (98.8 to 99.5)	97.5 (95.9 to 98.5)	99.7 (99.9 to 99.5)	97.1 (98.2 to 95.1)	92.5 (91.5 to 93.5)	71.4 (67.8 to 74.7)
3–5	96.9 (96.2 to 97.5)	93.3 (91.7 to 94.6)	98.6 (99.0 to 98.1)	91.6 (93.4 to 89.5)	90.2 (89.0 to 91.3)	59.7 (56.7 to 62.7)
6–10	90.4 (88.4 to 92.0)	83.4 (79.6 to 86.6)	93.4 (94.9 to 91.5)	79.1 (83.1 to 74.3)	78.7 (75.9 to 81.2)	42.0 (37.4 to 46.5)

Figure 2.
CAPRA scores and associated endpoint predictions [10].

PSA at Diagnosis (ng/mL)		Gleason Score at Biopsy (Primary/Secondary pattern)		Age at Diagnosis (Years)		Clinical Tumor Stage		% of Biopsy Cores Positive for Cancer	
<6.0	0	1–3/1–3	0	<50	0	T1a-T2c	0	≤33	0
6.0–10	1	1–3/4–5	1	≥50	1	T3a	1	>33	1
10.01–20	2	4–5/1–3	3						
20.01–30	3								
>30	4								

Table 2.
Calculating CAPRA scores.

made in coordination with physicians who have a longitudinal assessment of the patient, such as the primary medical doctor and cardiologist.

6. Imaging for prostate cancer

6.1 MRI imaging

Magnetic resonance imaging (MRI) is an essential modality for both staging and planning treatment, as it enables enhanced soft tissue resolution over computed tomography (CT). Multi-parametric MRI (mpMRI) includes standard MRI images obtained with at least one additional sequence such as diffusion-weighted imaging (DWI) or dynamic contrast-enhanced (DCE) images in addition to anatomic T2-weighted images. This imaging modality has aided in prostate cancer detection and risk stratification, has been widely used in patients who have a rising PSA with negative biopsies, and in patients who are undergoing active surveillance [12]. Due to its essential role for EBRT treatment, especially for high-dose stereotactic body radiation therapy (SBRT), if a patient is unable to obtain an MRI or his MRI imaging is suboptimal due to issues such as implanted metallic hardware, other treatment modalities such as prostatectomy or brachytherapy may be considered, as appropriate.

6.2 PSMA pet/CT

Several recent clinical trials have demonstrated the diagnostic and therapeutic benefits of prostate-specific membrane antigen (PSMA) in positron emission tomography (PET) imaging. The PSMA peptide is a transmembrane glycoprotein primarily expressed along the extracellular surface of the prostate cancer cell, enabling small molecule binding. The binding site serves as a target for biomarkers for both diagnostic and therapeutic purposes [13]. PSMA demonstrates 100-1000x greater overexpression in prostate adenocarcinoma cells compared to benign prostate tissue, which aids in detecting malignancy [14]. The proPSMA trial demonstrated increased sensitivity with PSMA PET/CT scan in identifying nodal metastatic prostate adenocarcinoma compared to conventional imaging, including the combined findings of CT and bone scans [15].

Both gallium-68 (68 Ga)-PSMA-11 (gozetotide) and fluorine-18 (18 F)-based PSMA compounds are currently widely in use for PET/CT imaging, and PSMA imaging has led to significant changes in clinical management. For example, in the CONDOR trial investigating the use of 18 F-DCFPy (Pylarify®, piflufolastat) in patients suspected to have a biochemical recurrence after prostatectomy or radiotherapy, among the 208 patients enrolled in the trial, the authors reported a 63.9% rate of change in management [16].

The SPOTLIGHT trial was presented at the American Urological Association Conference, which studied 18F-rhPSMA-7.3 in the biochemical recurrence setting in patients with elevated PSAs. All patients had negative results on conventional imaging, as read by three radiologists; however, on exploratory analysis, this radiotracer led to a 45–47% rate of upstaging [17].

7. Treatment for clinically localized disease

Evaluation of prostate cancer begins with a history and physical (H&P), assessing for baseline urinary function (e.g., American Urological Association [AUA] score/ International Prostate Symptom Score [IPSS]); sexual function (Sexual Health Inventory for Men [SHIM] score); bowel function; and prostate abnormalities on digital rectal examination (DRE) such as enlargement, induration, nodularity, extracapsular extension, and/or invasion. PSA and velocity (doubling time) should be calculated, and a prostate biopsy should be obtained, if not already.

7.1 Treatment options

This chapter discusses radiotherapy options for prostate adenocarcinoma, and will not delve into radical prostatectomy/surgical options. Potential radiotherapy options include photon EBRT, proton EBRT, and brachytherapy; EBRT includes standard fractionation (about nine weeks), moderate hypofractionation (about 4–5 weeks), or SBRT (about 4–5 sessions, recommended every other day to reduce toxicities). Intensity-modulated radiotherapy/image-guided radiotherapy (IMRT/IGRT) is strongly recommended to enable dose escalation, while reducing genitourinary (GU) and gastrointestinal (GI) toxicities. Fiducial markers are strongly recommended for

SBRT due to the extreme level of precision required and low number of fractions, and potentially for other EBRT treatments [8]; hydrogel spacers between the prostate and rectum may also be important for SBRT and brachytherapy to reduce the rectal dose, and in certain other EBRT cases [8].

Compared to conventional fractionation, moderate hypofractionation has demonstrated similar efficacy and toxicity in randomized trials, such as the CHHIP and PROFIT trials [18, 19]; however, some trials such as the HYPRO trial have demonstrated worse toxicity [20]. An ASTRO/ASCO/AUA evidence-based guideline concluded that hypofractionation is justified for routine use in this setting [21]. Common moderate hypofractionation regimens in the United States include 70 Gy/28 fractions, 70.2 Gy/26 fractions, and 60 Gy/20 fractions.

SBRT delivers highly-conformal, high-dose radiation in typically 4–5 fractions. Most of the data supporting SBRT are phase 2 trials demonstrating excellent biochemical progression-free survival and similar early toxicity to standard radiotherapy, but one phase 3 trial demonstrates non-inferiority of SBRT [22, 23]. Better candidates for SBRT have lower IPSS scores and prostates that are not significantly enlarged. SBRT with elective nodal irradiation is being explored, such as in the SATURN trial [24]. As well, SBRT is also being investigated as a neoadjuvant therapy before radical prostatectomy in high-risk patients, with phase I trials showing feasibility and safety, though one recent phase I trial assessing maximum tolerable dose was stopped early due to unacceptable toxicity [25, 26]. Additionally, some trials are looking at boosting the dominant intra-prostatic lesions to higher doses [27].

Brachytherapy monotherapy may be offered in the form of low-dose rate (LDR) or high-dose rate (HDR) brachytherapy. Alternatively, brachytherapy may be used as a boost after EBRT to 45–50.4 Gy for UIR, high-risk, and very high-risk prostate adenocarcinoma.

Proton radiotherapy has not demonstrated clear superior or inferior outcomes or differences in toxicity over photon radiotherapy, though one large Surveillance, Epidemiology, and End Results (SEER) study did demonstrate increased bowel toxicity [28]. Of note, proton therapy for prostate cancer is typically several times the cost of IMRT/IGRT treatments. The NCCN recommends proton therapy as a potential alternative to photon EBRT. Clinical trials are ongoing.

8. Very low- and low-risk prostate cancer

Patients with an NCCN risk-stratified very low- or low-risk prostate cancer and a life expectancy >10 years are usually recommended active surveillance (AS) [8]. This option involves obtaining a PSA no more often than every 6 months, DRE no more often than every 12 months, repeat biopsy no more often than yearly unless clinically indicated, and consideration of repeat mpMRIs no more often than every 12 months. Patients on AS are usually recommended curative-intent therapy if there is an increase in Gleason grade on repeat biopsy, tumor volume, or PSA density. Patient anxiety is also an important factor in management decisions, as patients may elect to come off of AS.

For patients with localized very low- or low-risk prostate cancer and a life expectancy of <5–10 years, observation ("watchful waiting") is generally recommended [8]. This process involves monitoring with a H&P and PSA no more often than every 12 months without biopsies until symptoms develop, or are thought to be imminent. Therapy is palliative only.

Per the NCCN guidelines, EBRT, proton therapy, SBRT, and brachytherapy monotherapy are potential radiotherapy treatment options for very low- and low-risk prostate cancer [8].

8.1 Favorable intermediate-risk (FIR) prostate cancer

Patients with FIR prostate cancer and a life expectancy >10–20 years are usually recommended curative-intent therapy [8]. However, active surveillance may be offered if there are more favorable tumor characteristics, significant co-morbidities, poor urinary function, and/or strong patient preference; patient compliance is important if active surveillance is chosen.

Per the NCCN guidelines, EBRT, proton therapy, SBRT, and brachytherapy monotherapy are potential radiotherapy treatment options for FIR [8].

8.2 Unfavorable intermediate risk (UIR) prostate cancer

UIR prostate cancer has been demonstrated to have an increased risk of pelvic and distant metastases versus FIR disease, and additional metastatic work-up is recommended, including either a CT abdomen/pelvis plus bone scan or alternatively a PSMA PET/CT [8, 9]. Treatment is recommended for those patients with >10 years life expectancy, while patients with <10 years are recommended observation. Brachytherapy may be offered as a boost, per the ASCENDE-RT trial, which demonstrated a significant difference at 10 years in biochemical disease-free survival, though no difference in OS and with more toxicities [29]; some researchers extrapolate that an overall survival (OS) difference may be reached with the passage of more time in this study.

Neoadjuvant, concurrent, and adjuvant short-term ADT is recommended in addition to radiotherapy in the form of a leutinizing hormone-releasing hormone agonist (e.g., goserelin or leuprolide) or antagonist (e.g., degarelix or relugolix) [8]. This recommendation is based on a modest but significant improvement in OS at 10 years in UIR patients receiving short-term ADT [30, 31]. ADT is usually initiated 2 months before RT, though the sequencing is subject to change. It is hypothesized that ADT radiosensitizes prostate cancer by decreasing non-homologous end-joining DNA repair, thereby acting synergistically with radiotherapy. ADT may also shrink the prostate and primary tumor, which may theoretically decrease the target volume and GI/GU toxicities. With combination EBRT/brachytherapy boost for UIR prostate cancer, short-term ADT may be omitted [8].

Per the NCCN guidelines, EBRT, proton therapy, SBRT, and combination EBRT/brachytherapy are potential radiotherapy treatment options for UIR [8].

9. High-risk and very high-risk prostate cancer

For high- and very-high risk prostate cancer, curative intent treatment is recommended for men with life expectancies >5 years or who are symptomatic, whereas men asymptomatic with <5 years life expectancy may be managed with observation, ADT alone, or EBRT alone [8]. With the publication of the POP-RT study incorporating Pylarify PET/CTs, the authors recommend treating the pelvic lymph nodes, as the arm treating the pelvic lymph nodes had improved 5-year disease-free survival over the prostate-only arm of 89.5% vs. 77.2% ($p = 0.002$) [32]. The NRG now recommends that for pelvic lymph node treatments, the superior border starts at L5-S1 and extends to L4-L5 [33]. Long-term ADT for 1.5–3 years is recommended based on an OS benefit demonstrated with long-term ADT over RT alone or short-term ADT [34–36].

Per the NCCN guidelines, EBRT, proton therapy, SBRT, and combination EBRT/brachytherapy are potential radiotherapy treatment options for high-risk and very high-risk prostate adenocarcinoma [8]. However, the authors wish to comment that treating the prostate/seminal vesicles with SBRT alone, and not addressing the lymph nodes, may conflict with the results of the POP-RT study, in which addressing the pelvic lymph nodes demonstrated a disease-free survival benefit [32].

10. Adjuvant and early salvage radiotherapy

Unfortunately, 20–50% of patients may experience either biochemical recurrence or a persistently-elevated PSA within 5–10 years after prostatectomy [37]. Three randomized trials established the benefit of adjuvant radiotherapy, which improved the 10-year biochemical recurrence-free survival to about 60% from about 30–40% [38]. There has been ongoing debate as to the timing of radiotherapy, i.e. whether it should be delivered in the adjuvant setting (within 12–16 weeks post-prostatectomy while PSA remains undetectable) or as salvage radiotherapy (initiated in the presence of detectable PSA or a palpable nodule on DRE). The ARTISTIC meta-analysis found that adjuvant RT did not improve the 5-year event free survival over salvage radiotherapy in localized or locally-advanced disease, supporting the use of early salvage treatment [39].

The decision of whether to treat should include risk stratification based on multiple factors such as age, co-morbidities, size/number of positive margin(s), the absolute PSA level, PSA doubling time, nomograms, and molecular assays (e.g., Decipher® Score). Given conflicting conclusions in studies comparing adjuvant versus salvage radiotherapy, the NCCN recommends curative intent adjuvant or early salvage radiotherapy in patients with life expectancies >5 years with detectable PSA and adverse pathologic features (e.g., positive margins, seminal vesical invasion or extra-prostatic extension), or positive nodes [8]. The work-up for post-operative patients with evidence of persistent or recurrent disease includes H&P, DRE, PSA, MRI, and PSMA PET/CT (preferred over CT plus bone scan, per NCCN 2023 update), consecutive PSA measurements ≥0.2 ng/ml, and potentially a biopsy of the prostate bed.

The ASTRO/AUA guidelines recommend at least 64–65 Gy in the post-operative setting, with no distinction between adjuvant and salvage treatment [40]. Hypofractionated regimens in the adjuvant and salvage setting are currently being investigated. Three phase 2 trials utilized regimens of 65 Gy/26 fractions, 54 Gy/18 fractions, and 51 Gy/17 fractions, and demonstrated excellent efficacy and low rates of toxicity [41–43]. The NRG-GU003 phase 3 trial is randomizing patients to conventional fractionation (66.6 Gy/37) vs. hypofractionation (62.5 Gy/25 fx); it is currently closed to accrual, with expected completion in 2026 [44].

The RTOG 96–01 trial assessed the addition of 24 months of bicalutamide to radiotherapy in patients with biochemical failure, and demonstrated improved 12-year OS in salvage patients with PSA >0.61 ng/mL, but men with PSA ≤ 0.6 ng/mL (i.e., early salvage patients) experienced increased other-cause mortality and cardiac events [45]. The GETUG-AFU 16 trial assessed the addition of 6 months of ADT for patients with biochemical failure; at 120 months, the progression-free survival was

64% for patients with radiotherapy plus goserelin and 49% for patients with radiotherapy alone (HR = 0.54, p < 0.0001) [46]. The NRG Oncology/RTOG 05–34 SPPORT trial has demonstrated an improved 5-year freedom from progression with the addition of ADT to prostate bed radiotherapy (PBRT) over PBRT alone, 81% vs. 71% [47]. The SPPORT trial is also assessing the addition of pelvic nodal radiotherapy to PBRT+ADT, and demonstrated an improved 5-year freedom from progression (87%) versus the groups mentioned above. Acute toxicities are significantly worse with the addition of ADT and with ADT + pelvic nodal radiotherapy, but no differences were seen in late toxicities.

The NCCN now recommends obtaining the Decipher® molecular assay to help individualize treatment decisions in the post-operative setting; patients with a high Decipher® genomic classifier Score (>0.6) should be strongly considered for EBRT with ADT in patients who have not received early salvage therapy [8].

11. Approach to a patient with a rising PSA after radiotherapy

Following definitive therapy for prostate adenocarcinoma, the NCCN recommends obtaining a PSA every 6–12 months for 5 years, and then annually thereafter [8]. As well, a PSA may be obtained as frequently as every 3 months to clarify disease status in certain cases, especially for patients with aggressive disease. PSA failure post-radiotherapy is defined by the Phoenix Consensus as a PSA increase by 2 ng/mL or more above the nadir. A work-up for recurrence can begin prior to reaching nadir +2 ng/mL, especially for candidates for salvage treatments with long life expectancies, and if there is a rapid increase in the PSA. However, it is important to note that many patients do experience 1–2 PSA upward "bounces" that resolve. There are data demonstrating that a PSA nadir >0.5 ng/mL is associated with lower rates of biochemical control, distant metastasis-free survival, prostate cancer specific survival, and OS [48].

Work-up in the setting of current or impending biochemical failure includes PSMA imaging, MRI-prostate, and testosterone. Prostate biopsy is required for confirmation of recurrence, especially if local salvage therapy (e.g., high-dose rate [HDR] brachytherapy, low-dose rate [HDR] brachytherapy, SBRT, radical prostatectomy, high intensity focused ultrasound, or cryotherapy) is desired.

NRG Oncology/RTOG 0526 prospectively analyzed patients who had prior EBRT and experienced local failure, and were treated with salvage LDR [49]. This study included patients treated with EBRT for low- or intermediate-risk prostate adenocarcinoma with EBRT and biopsy-proven local failure >30 months after definitive treatment. Inclusion criteria also included PSA <10 ng/mL, and no regional/distant disease. Between May 2007–January 2014, 20 centers administered salvage treatment to 100 patients, of whom 92 patients were analyzable. The median prior EBRT dose was 74 Gy, and median follow-up was 6.7 years, with LDR administered at a median time of 85 months after EBRT. ADT was combined with salvage radiotherapy for only 16% of patients. Ten-year OS was 70%, with disease-free survival of 61% at 5 years and 33% at 10 years; of note, local failure was rare at 5% at 10 years.

A meta-analysis was performed of salvage treatments after definitive radiotherapy, consisting of 150 studies, seeking to compare the efficacy and toxicity of the six techniques listed above (HDR, LDR, SBRT, radical prostatectomy, high intensity focused ultrasound, and cryotherapy) [50]. HDR brachytherapy and SBRT had the highest rates of adjusted 5-year recurrence free-survival at 60%, while cryotherapy had the lowest at 50%. CTCAE grade ≥ 3 GU toxicity was the lowest for SBRT at 4.2%, and the highest for HIFU at 23%; as well, CTCAE grade ≥ 3 GI toxicity was the lowest for SBRT and HDR at 0.0%, and the highest for radical prostatectomy at 1.9%. From this retrospective meta-analysis, the authors concluded that the radiotherapy techniques appeared most effective in reducing recurrence and limiting severe GU toxicity; severe GI toxicity remained low regardless of technique.

12. Evaluation for treatment of oligo-metastatic and poly-metastatic disease

When a patient presents with a metastatic focus (or foci) after prior definitive treatment, the decision for a biopsy is often not answerable by a straightforward algorithm. The clinical situation as a whole has to be evaluated. Some pertinent questions include:

- What was the original NCCN risk category? What were the Gleason score, volume of disease, pre-treatment PSA, MRI findings, and DRE findings?
- On the pre-treatment work-up/imaging, were any abnormalities noted on the suspicious focus/foci?
- What is the current PSA? Is the patient currently on ADT?
- What is the size of the lesion and its SUV on PSMA PET/CT?
- How many lesions are there?
- Is the focus actually the ureter(s) (very common conflation with a positive lymph node on PSMA PET/CT readings)?
- Is the focus accessible to biopsy?

These questions may be best addressed in a multi-disciplinary setting, such as a Genitourinary Tumor Board. As well, shared decision-making regarding the risks/benefits and logistics of a biopsy with the patient is important.

Numerous studies have provided insight into the value of treating the primary site and/or metastatic sites for prostate adenocarcinoma. The HORRAD trial from the Netherlands was a multi-center randomized controlled trial to determine whether OS is prolonged by adding prostate EBRT to ADT for patients with metastatic prostate adenocarcinoma [51]. From 2004 to 2014, the study recruited 432 patients with a PSA >20 ng/mL and metastatic prostate adenocarcinoma on bone scan. The patients were then randomized to either ADT with EBRT (radiotherapy group) or ADT alone (control group). OS was the primary endpoint, and PSA progression was the secondary endpoint. In this trial, the median PSA was 142 ng/mL, and 67% of patients had >5 osseous metastases. At a median follow-up of 47 months, the median OS was 45 months in the radiotherapy group and 43 months in the ADT alone group, which was not statistically significant (HR = 0.90, CI = 0.70–1.14, p = 0.4). There was a benefit in time to PSA progression for the radiotherapy group of 15 months versus 12 months (HR = 0.78, CI = 0.63–0.97, p = 0.02).

On a subgroup analysis of 160 patients with <5 bone metastases, an OS benefit started to emerge with HR = 0.68 (CI = 0.42–1.10). However, in this study, the number of bone metastases were categorized as 1–4, 5–15, and > 15; the authors postulated that an upper cut-off of 1–3 metastases may have been statistically significant for the radiotherapy group for OS.

The "Systemic Therapy in Advancing or Metastatic Prostate Cancer: Evaluation of Drug Efficacy" (STAMPEDE) trial studied if local radiotherapy to the prostate would improve OS in men with metastatic prostate adenocarcinoma, with the benefit greatest in men with a low metastatic burden [52]. This study randomized 2061 patients in a 1:1 ratio to standard of care (control group) or standard of care and radiotherapy (radiotherapy group). Standard of care consisted of lifelong ADT, with up-front docetaxel allowed starting from December 2015. The radiotherapy arm received either 55 Gy/20 fractions over 4 weeks, or 36 Gy/6 fractions over 6 weeks. Overall, radiotherapy to the prostate did not improve OS for unselected patients; however, within the subgroup that had a low metastatic burden (non-regional lymph nodes or ≤ 3 bone metastases without visceral metastases), local radiotherapy to the prostate did confer an OS advantage of 65% vs. 53% at 5 years (HR = 0.64, $p < 0.001$) [53].

Radiotherapy to the prostate was not recommended for patients with high-volume metastatic disease unless in the context of a clinical trial or for palliative intent. The concern was that this aggressive treatment would increase toxicity, without a meaningful effect on OS. Of note, many experts would argue that the definition of low-volume disease should not be applied to metastases only detected on Pylarify PET/CT (and not on bone scan/conventional CT), since this imaging modality was not used in the STAMPEDE trial, and will detect smaller metastases.

The "Observation versus Stereotactic Ablative Radiation for Oligometastatic Prostate Cancer" (ORIOLE) phase II randomized trial studied whether SBRT to the oligometastases improves oncologic outcomes for men with oligometastatic prostate adenocarcinoma, and may thereby delay initiation of ADT [54]. The study randomized 54 men with recurrent hormone-sensitive prostate cancer and 1–3 metastases detectable by conventional imaging in a 2:1 ratio to receive SBRT or observation. SBRT improved median progression-free survival (not reached vs. 5.8 months, HR = 0.30, $p = 0.02$), and the risk of progression at 6 months from 61–19%. There were no acute grade ≥ 3 toxicities.

Data from the ORIOLE trial appeared to indicate that sub-total metastasis-directed therapy (MDT) is not beneficial in extending progression-free survival. In this study, the treating radiation oncologists did not have access to PSMA PET/CT, and treated based upon conventional imaging; therefore, within the SBRT arm (36 patients), 16 patients actually had untreated lesions. The progression-free survival was 63% at 6 months in the sub-total consolidation arm, which was similar to the observation arm (61%). The authors concluded that MDT of all radiotracer-avid disease could potentially provide excellent progression-free survival for oligo-metastatic disease, with limited acute toxicity.

As well, the "Surveillance or Metastasis-Directed Therapy for Oligometastatic Prostate Cancer Recurrence: A Prospective, Randomized, Multicenter Phase II Trial" (STOMP) study also analyzed the benefit of MDT in a randomized phase II trial [55]. The trial included patients with asymptomatic prostate cancer with a biochemic recurrence after primary treatment, 1–3 extracranial metastatic lesions, and serum testosterone levels >50 ng/mL (non-castrate level). Sixty-two patients were randomly assigned at 1:1 to either surveillance or MDT of all lesions, with local therapy including surgery or SBRT. At a median follow-up time of 3 years, the median ADT-free survival was 13 months for the surveillance group, versus 21 months for the MDT group. Quality-of-life measures were similar between the two arms at baseline, as well as at 3 months and 12 months; there were no grade 2–5 toxicities. The STOMP study also concluded that MDT increases progression-free survival, as well as ADT-free survival.

A recent non-randomized, prospective phase II trial incorporated PSMA PET/CT-staged patients for confirmation of oligometastatic disease after local curative treatment (surgery and/or radiotherapy), and to demonstrate the efficacy and safety of "local ablative radiotherapy" (*authors' designation, though many patients received the non-ablative fractionation of 50 Gy/25 fractions*) [56]. The OLI-P study used gallium-68 PSMA PET/CT to stage patients at two German cancer centers between 2014 and 2018. Patients with ≤5 PSMA PET-positive bone (OSS-MET) or lymph node (LN-MET) metastases without local tumor recurrence or visceral metastases were included in the trial; as well, they must have had no ongoing ADT, PSA <10 ng/mL, and life expectancy ≥5 years. Fractionation schedules were either 30 Gy/3 fractions (stereotactic) or 50 Gy/25 fractions (conventional). The primary endpoint was treatment-related toxicity (grade ≥ 2) at 24 months after the start of local ablative radiotherapy; second endpoints included PSA progression-free time (event defined as initial PSA value +20%, or the start of ADT), progression-free survival (event defined as PSA progression, start of ADT, distant progression, or death), and OS.

A total of 72 patients were recruited, with 63 patients receiving local ablative radiotherapy; five patients were later determined to not fulfill the inclusion criteria, and for another four patients, a decision was made during radiotherapy planning not to proceed due to a very significant overlap with prior radiotherapy fields for the primary tumor. The study's median follow-up time was 37.2 months. There were 68 LN-METS and 21 OSS-METS treated; of note, most patients (n = 45, 71%) only had one lesion.

During follow-up, there were no treatment-related grade ≥ 2 adverse events by two years after local ablative radiotherapy. Regarding secondary endpoints, the median time to PSA progression was 13.2 months, progression-free survival was 21.4% at 3 years, and OS was 94.6% at 3 years. The authors concluded that local ablative radiotherapy was a safe and an effective option for selected patients to delay systemic therapy.

In view of the data, the ESTRO-ACROP Delphi consensus published the following four recommendations in *Radiotherapy & Oncology* in October 2022: [57].

- PSMA PET imaging is the preferred staging and restaging imaging modality for oligometastatic, oligorecurrent, and oligoprogressive prostate cancer patients

- Metastasis-directed radiotherapy (MDRT) may be considered for patients diagnosed with up to 5 lymph nodal, bone, or visceral metastases in all disease settings

- Systemic therapy with loco-regional irradiation and MDRT of all metastatic lesions is the preferred option for synchronous *de novo* oligometastatic hormone-sensitive patients

- MDRT of all lesions without switch of systemic therapy is recommended for patients with oligoprogressive castration-resistant prostate cancer

Ongoing phase III trials for MDT include the following, in **Table 3** [58–62].

Study	Name	Primary Objective
NCT02759783	Conventional Care Versus Radioablation (Stereotactic Body Radiotherapy) for Extracranial Oligometastases	Progression-free survival at 60 months post-treatment; time from randomization to evidence of progression of cancer at any site or death from any cause; includes prostate, breast, and non-small cell lung cancer primary tumors
NCT02685397	Management of Castration-Resistant Prostate Cancer with Oligometastases (PCS IX)	Radiographic progression-free survival, or the start of new anti-neoplastic therapy
NCT02274779	Salvage Radiotherapy Combined with Hormonotherapy in Oligometastatic Pelvic Node Relapses of Prostate Cancer (OLIGOPELVIS)	Biochemical or clinical relapse-free survival at 2 years
NCT03143322	Standard Treatment +/− SBRT in Solid Tumors Patients with Between 1 and 3 Bone-Only Metastases (STEREO-OS)	Progression-free survival (to evaluate the impact of SBRT on progression-free survival at 1 year according to RECIST 1.1 and PERCIST 1.0 criteria)
NCT03569241	PEACE V: Salvage Treatment of OligoRecurrent Nodal Prostate Cancer Metastases (STORM)	Metastasis-free survival

Table 3.
Ongoing prospective trials for metastasis-directed therapy.

13. Prostate genomics

The six-tier NCCN risk group classification system provides a highly-validated basic framework for standard treatment recommendations [8]. However, a variety of advanced risk stratification tools have been developed and are in various stages of validation that independently improve stratification. The NCCN recommends ordering these tests for borderline cases as an extra data point that may potentially change management; patients with low-risk, favorable intermediate-risk, unfavorable intermediate-risk, and high-risk tumors with a life expectancy ≥10 years may be candidates for Decipher®, Oncotype Dx Prostate®, or Prolaris® [63]. Indeed, research has demonstrated that the current risk stratification systems are frequently poor prognosticators for clinically-meaningful endpoints; for distant metastases rates at 10-years, the concordance index (c-index) for the NCCN classification system was 0.73 (95% CI, 0.60–0.86) and for CAPRA was 0.74 (95% CI, 0.65–0.84) [64]. Per the NCCN, Decipher® currently has the highest level of evidence for validation among the major genomic classifiers (GCs), having been validated in the context of multiple clinical trials with consistent results (see **Table 4**) [63].

Numerous studies have been performed, and are ongoing, to validate GCs. One notable example includes validation of the 22-gene Decipher® GC from the biobank from the phase III randomized trial NRG Oncology/RTOG 0126 [64]. This trial compared men with intermediate-risk prostate cancer randomized to 70.2 Gy versus 79.2 Gy, without androgen deprivation therapy. RNA was extracted from the highest grade tumor foci, and for 215 patients (of the 1532 patients in the study), the material passed quality control. GC data were generated and compared to the patients' respective clinical outcomes on the study, for a retrospective analysis of the prospective trial. The GC proved independently prognostic for disease progression ($p = 0.03$),

Genomic Classifier	Level of Evidence for Validation
Decipher®	1
Prolaris®	3
Oncotype®	3

Level 1: Validation in the context of multiple clinical trials with consistent results.
Level 2: Validation in multiple prospective registry/observational cohorts with consistent results.
Level 3: Validation in multiple independent retrospective studies with consistent results.
Level 4: Validation in a single retrospective study, or multiple independent retrospective studies with inconsistent results.

Table 4.
Levels of evidence for major prostate genomic classifiers [8].

biochemical failure ($p < 0.001$), distant metastasis ($p = 0.01$), and prostate cancer-specific mortality ($p < 0.001$). The authors deemed that the GC can be used to help personalize treatment for intermediate-risk prostate adenocarcinoma.

In 2021, prostate cancer researchers published "A Systematic Review of the Evidence for the Decipher Genomic Classifier in Prostate Cancer" in *European Urology* [65]. This systematic review incorporated 42 studies and 30,407 patients with localized, post-prostatectomy, non-metastatic castration-resistant, or metastatic hormone-sensitive prostate adenocarcinoma. The patients were part of retrospective studies (n = 12,141), prospective registries (n = 17,053), and prospective and post-hoc randomized trial analyses (n = 1213). For 32 studies, the GC proved independently prognostic for all study endpoints (adverse pathology, biochemical failure, metastasis-free survival, cancer-specific survival, and OS) on multi-variate analysis, and improved discrimination over the standard of care in 24 studies. As well, the GC changed management for the AS (NNT = 9) and post-prostatectomy (NNT = 1.5–4) settings. Its utility was deemed strongest for decision-making with intermediate-risk prostate adenocarcinoma and post-prostatectomy. Indeed, despite the ongoing debates about adjuvant and salvage radiotherapy in the setting of adverse pathologic risk factors without biochemical failure, the NCCN Prostate Guidelines now (Version 1.2023) recommends that Decipher® "should be considered if not previously performed to inform adjuvant treatment if adverse features are found post-RP;" [63] as well, as discussed previously, the NCCN recommends strongly considering post-prostatectomy radiotherapy and ADT when the Decipher® GC score is high (>0.6) [63].

A clinical-genomic model has been developed that incorporates the NCCN risk groups with the Decipher® GC, thereby creating a clinical-genomic point system. This model has an improved c-index of 0.84 (95% CI, 0.61–0.93), versus 0.73 (95% CI, 0.60–0.86) for the NCCN six-tiered classification system alone (see **Figure 3**) [64].

Regarding patients on AS, several studies have demonstrated the utility of GCs in determining which patients would have biopsy reclassification on serial biopsies, and therefore stop AS in favor of definitive treatment. A study at the University of California, San Francisco studied men with clinically low-risk prostate cancer prospectively enrolled on AS between 2000 and 2016 [66]. In this study, biopsy re-classification was defined as Gleason grade group ≥2 on subsequent biopsy. On multi-variate analysis, biopsy re-classification at 3–5 years was strongly associated with a high genomic score (HR = 2.81); it was also strongly associated with a PSA density ≥ 0.15 (HR = 3.37), rapid PSA kinetics (HR = 2.19), and percentage biopsy cores positive (HR = 1.27). Of note, a PI-RADS 4–5 score on MRI was not associated with

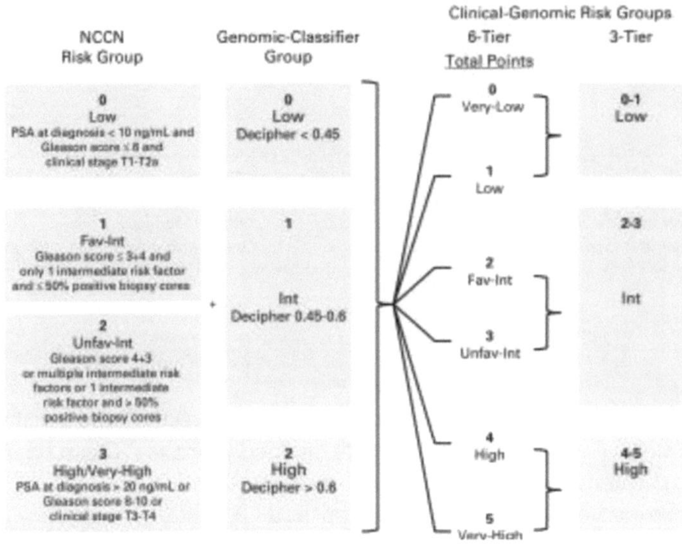

Figure 3.
Clinical-genomic point system using a genomic classifier [63, 64].

biopsy re-classification. In a multi-institutional study led by the University of Michigan, 855 men underwent Decipher® testing of their prostate biopsies between February 2015–October 2019, of whom 264 (31%) proceeded with AS [67]. For the men who chose AS, after adjusting for NCCN risk group and all risk factors, a high-risk Decipher® score was independently associated with a shorter time to treatment failure (HR = 2.51, $p < 0.001$). Of note, for the men who proceeded with radical therapy, a high Decipher® score was independently associated with a shorter time to treatment failure on multi-variate analysis.

Numerous prospective trials are currently ongoing to evaluate the effectiveness of these markers, and to better assess their utility for enhancing risk stratification, including the following studies, as demonstrated in **Table 5** [68–70].

Additionally, while the usage of artificial intelligence is still an NCCN category IIB recommendation at this time for aiding with risk stratification, new studies suggest it will have an increasing role in cancer therapy precision [8, 71].

14. Summary

The evaluation of patients who have been diagnosed with prostate adenocarcinoma is a changing paradigm, and an important one for an extremely prevalent, but often non-aggressive malignancy. Since the advent of PSA testing, patients are usually diagnosed at earlier stages, often creating the difficult questions of who needs to be treated, when, and how aggressively. As well, patient evaluation is important in the adjuvant and locally-recurrent scenarios. With increasing data on treating oligometastatic cancers, local treatment and MDT are increasingly supported by data and utilized to improve cancer endpoints. Enhanced imaging, such as PSMA PET/CT, is improving the sensitivity of detecting metastases and recurrent disease, and thereby helping in patient selection and ensuring meaningful local treatment and MDT, given the potential for toxicity.

Study	Name	Primary Objective
NRG Oncology GU-009	Parallel Phase III Randomized Trials or High Risk Prostate Cancer Evaluating De-Intensification For Lower Genomic Risk and Intensification of Concurrent Therapy for Higher Genomic Risk with Radiation (Predict-RT*) *Prostate RNA Expression/Decipher To Individualize Concurrent Therapy with Radiation	De-Intensification Study: To determine whether men with NCCN high-risk prostate cancer who are in the lower 2/3 of Decipher genomic risk (≤0.85) can be treated with 12 months of ADT plus RT instead of 24 months ADT + RT and experience non-inferior metastasis-free survival Intensification Study: To determine whether men with NCCN high-risk prostate cancer who are in the upper 1/3 of Decipher genomic risk (>0.85) or have node-positive disease by conventional imaging (MRI or CT scan) will have a superior metastasis-free survival (MFS) through treatment intensification with apalutamide added to the standard of RT plus 24 months of ADT
NRG Oncology GU-010	Parallel Phase III Randomized Trials of Genomic-Risk Stratified Unfavorable Intermediate Risk Prostate Cancer: De-Intensification and Intensification Clinical Trial Evaluation (Guidance)	De-Intensification Study: To determine whether men with unfavorable intermediate-risk prostate cancer and lower Decipher genomic risk (<0.40) treated with RT alone instead of 6 months ADT + RT experience non-inferior rate of distant metastasis Intensification Study: To determine whether men with unfavorable intermediate-risk prostate cancer who are in the higher genomic risk (Decipher score ≥ 0.40) will have a superior metastasis-free survival through treatment intensification with darolutamide added to the standard of RT plus 6 months of ADT
NCT 04396808	Genomics in Michigan to AdJust Outcomes in Prostate cancer (G-MAJOR) for Men with Newly Diagnosed Favorable Risk Prostate Cancer	Binomial proportion of men on active surveillance without treatment at 2 years (studies active surveillance with genomic classifiers including Decipher®, Prolaris®, and Oncotype Dx®)

Table 5.
Ongoing prospective trials for validation of genomic classifiers.

The NCCN Prostate Panel itself acknowledges that the six-tier classification system has limited predictive/prognostic value, which has been confirmed in studies, and it recommends additional studies for borderline cases. GCs have demonstrated significant prognostic value, and are undergoing increasing validation in numerous studies. As medicine increasingly progresses from personalized medicine to precision medicine, and GCs' prospective studies have an opportunity for maturation of their data, GCs will very likely have a much more significant impact on patient evaluation and ensuring the most appropriate treatment regimens.

Author details

Jonathan B. Wallach*, Chana Stern, Michael Karp and David L. Schwartz
Department of Radiation Oncology, VA New York Harbor Healthcare System, SUNY Downstate Medical Center, Brooklyn, NY, USA

*Address all correspondence to: wallach.jonathan@gmail.com

References

[1] Sung H, Ferlay J, Siegel RL, et al. Global cancer statistics 2020: GLOBOCAN estimates of incidence and mortality worldwide for 36 cancers in 185 countries. CA: A Cancer Journal for Clinicians. 2021;**71**(3):209-249

[2] Rawla P. Epidemiology of prostate cancer. World Journal of Oncology. 2019;**10**(2):63-89

[3] Giona S. Chapter 1: The epidemiology of prostate cancer. In: Bott SRJ, Ng KL, editors. Prostate Cancer. Brisbane (AU): Exon Publications; 2021

[4] Prostate Cancer: Screening. US Preventive Services Taskforce. Available from: https://www.uspreventiveservicestaskforce.org/uspstf/recommendation/prostate-cancer-screening [Accessed: November 23, 2022]

[5] American Cancer Society Recommendations for Prostate Cancer Early Detection. American Cancer Society. American Cancer Society Recommendations for Prostate Cancer Early Detection. Available from: https://www.cancer.org/cancer/prostate-cancer/detection-diagnosis-staging/acs-recommendations.html [Accessed: November 23, 2022]

[6] Epstein JI, Egevad L, Amin MB, Delahunt B, Srigley JR, Humphrey PA, et al. The 2014 International Society of Urological Pathology (ISUP) consensus conference on Gleason grading of prostatic carcinoma: Definition of grading patterns and proposal for a new grading system. The American Journal of Surgical Pathology. 2016;**40**(2):244-252

[7] D'Amico AV, Whittington R, Malkowicz SB, et al. Biochemical outcome after radical prostatectomy, external beam radiation therapy, or interstitial radiation therapy for clinically localized prostate cancer. Journal of the American Medical Association. 1998;**280**(11):969-974

[8] National Comprehensive Cancer Network®. NCCN Guidelines Version 1. 2023: Prostate Cancer. NCCN Clinical Practice Guidelines in Oncology (NCCN Guidelines ®). PROS-2, PROS-3, PROS-4, PROS-5, PROS-6, PROS-7, PROS-8, PROS-8A, PROS-9, PROS-10, PROS-D, PROG-G, MS-25. Plymouth Meeting, Pennsylvania: National Comprehensive Cancer Network®; 2022

[9] Zumsteg ZS, Spratt DE, Pei I, et al. A new risk classification system for therapeutic decision making with intermediate-risk prostate cancer patients undergoing dose-escalated external-beam radiation therapy. European Urology. 2013;**64**(6):895-902

[10] Cooperberg MR, Broering JM, Carroll PR. Risk assessment for prostate cancer metastasis and mortality at the time of diagnosis. Journal of the National Cancer Institute. 2009;**101**(12):878-887

[11] Prostate Cancer Nomograms. Memorial Sloan-Kettering Cancer Center. Available from: https://www.mskcc.org/nomograms/prostate. [Accessed: November 23, 2022]

[12] Demirel HC, Davis JW. Multiparametric magnetic resonance imaging: Overview of the technique, clinical applications in prostate biopsy and future directions. Turkish Journal of Urology. 2018;**44**(2):93-102

[13] Wright GL Jr, Haley C, Beckett ML, Schellhammer PF. Expression of prostate-specific membrane antigen in normal, benign, and malignant prostate tissues. Urologic Oncology. 1995;**1**(1): 18-28

[14] Jones W, Griffiths K, Barata PC, Paller CJ. PSMA Theranostics: Review of the current status of PSMA-targeted imaging and Radioligand therapy. Cancers (Basel). 2020;**12**(6):1367

[15] Hofman MS, Lawrentschuk N, Francis RJ, et al. Prostate-specific membrane antigen PET-CT in patients with high-risk prostate cancer before curative-intent surgery or radiotherapy (proPSMA): A prospective, randomised, multicentre study. Lancet. 2020; **395**(10231):1208-1216

[16] Kuo P, Hesterman J, Rahbar K, et al. [68Ga]Ga-PSMA-11 PET baseline imaging as a prognostic tool for clinical outcomes to [177Lu]Lu-PSMA-617 in patients with mCRPC: A VISION substudy. Clinical Oncology. 2022;**40** (suppl. 16):5002

[17] Imaging Study to Investigate Safety and Diagnostic Performance of rhPSMA 7.3 (18F) PET Ligand in Suspected Prostate Cancer Recurrence (SPOTLIGHT). Available from: Clinica lTrials.gov [Accessed: September 28, 2022]

[18] Dearnaley D, Syndikus I, Mossop H, et al. Conventional versus hypofractionated high-dose intensity-modulated radiotherapy for prostate cancer: 5-year outcomes of the randomized, non-inferiority, phase 3 CHHip trial. The Lancet Oncology. 2016; **17**(8):1047-1060

[19] Catton CN, Lukka H, Gu CS, et al. Randomized trial of a Hypofractionated radiation regimen for the treatment of localized prostate cancer. Journal of Clinical Oncology. 2017;**35**(17): 1884-1890

[20] Incrocci L, Wortel RC, Alemayehu WG, et al. Hypofractionated versus conventionally fractionated radiotherapy for patients with localized prostate cancer (HYPRO): Final efficacy results from a randomized, multicentre, open-label, phase 3 trial. The Lancet Oncology. 2016;**17**(8):1061-1069

[21] Morgan SC, Hoffman K, Loblaw DA, et al. Hypofractionated radiation therapy for localized prostate cancer: An ASTRO, ASCO, and AUA evidence-based guideline. Journal of Clinical Oncology. 2018;**36**(34):JCO1801097

[22] King CR, Freeman D, Kaplan I, et al. Stereotactic body radiotherapy for localized prostate cancer: Pooled analysis from a multi-institutional consortium of prospective phase II trials. Radiotherapy and Oncology. 2013;**109**(2):217-221

[23] Widmark A, Gunnlaugsson A, Beckman L, et al. Ultra-hypofractionated versus conventionally fractionated radiotherapy for prostate cancer: 5-year outcomes of the HYPO-RT-PC randomized, non-inferiority, phase 3 trial. Lancet. 2019;**394**(10196):385-395

[24] Musunuru HB, D'Alimonte L, Davidson M, et al. Phase 1-2 study of stereotactic ablative radiotherapy including regional lymph node irradiation in patients with high-risk prostate cancer (SATURN): Early toxicity and quality of life. IJROBP. 2018; **102**(5):1438-1447

[25] Parikh NR, Kishan AU, Kane N, et al. Phase 1 trial of stereotactic body radiation therapy Neoadjuvant to radical prostatectomy for patients with high-risk prostate cancer. IJROBP. 2020; **108**(4):930-935

[26] Hammer L, Jiang R, Hearn J, et al. A phase I trial of Neoadjuvant stereotactic body radiotherapy prior to radical prostatectomy for locally advanced prostate cancer. IJROBP. 2022;**115**: 132-141

[27] Draulans C, van der Heide UA, Haustermans K, et al. Primary endpoint analysis of the multicentre phase II hypo-FLAME trial for intermediate and high risk prostate cancer. Radiotherapy and Oncology. 2020;**147**:92-98

[28] Sheets NC, Goldin GH, Meyer AM, et al. Intensity-modulated radiation therapy, proton therapy, or conformal radiation therapy and morbidity and disease control in localized prostate cancer. Journal of the American Medical Association. 2012;**307**(15): 1611-1620

[29] Morris WJ, Tyldesley S, Rodda S, et al. Androgen suppression combined with elective nodal and dose escalated radiation therapy (the ASCENDE-RT trial): An analysis of survival endpoints for a randomized trial comparing a low-dose-rate brachytherapy boost to a dose-escalated external beam boost for high- and intermediate-risk prostate cancer. IJROBP. 2017;**98**(2):275-285

[30] Denham JW, Steigler A, Lamb DS, et al. Short-term neoadjuvant androgen deprivation and radiotherapy for locally advanced prostate cancer: 10-year data from the TROG 96.01 randomised trial. The Lancet Oncology. 2011;**12**(5): 451-459

[31] Jones CU, Pugh SL, Sandler HM, et al. Adding short-term androgen deprivation therapy to radiation therapy in men with localized prostate cancer: Long-term update of the NRG/RTOG 9408 randomized clinical trial. IJROBP. 2022;**112**(2):294-303

[32] Murthy V, Maitre P, Kannan S, et al. Prostate-only versus whole-pelvic radiation therapy in high-risk and very high-risk prostate cancer (POP-RT): Outcomes from phase III randomized controlled trial. Journal of Clinical Oncology. 2021;**39**(11):1234-1242

[33] Hall WA, Paulson E, Davis BJ, et al. NRG oncology updated international consensus atlas on pelvic lymph node volumes for intact and postoperative prostate cancer. IJROBP. 2021;**109**(1): 174-185

[34] Kishan AU, Sun Y, Hartman H, et al. Androgen deprivation therapy use and duration with definitive radiotherapy for localized prostate cancer: An individual patient data meta-analysis. The Lancet Oncology. 2022;**23**(2):304-316

[35] Bolla M, de Reijke TM, Van Tienhoven G, et al. Duration of androgen suppression in the treatment of prostate cancer. NEJM. 2009;**360**:2516-2527

[36] Bolla M, Collette L, Blank L, et al. Long-term results with immediate androgen suppression and external irradiation in patients with locally advanced prostate cancer (an EORTC study): A phase III randomized trial. Lancet. 2002;**360**(9327):103-106

[37] Stephenson AJ, Scardino PT, Eastham JA, et al. Preoperative nomogram predicting the 10-year probability of prostate cancer recurrence after radical prostatectomy. Journal of the National Cancer Institute. 2006; **98**(10):715-717

[38] Ko EC, Michaud AL, Valicenti RK. Postoperative radiation after radical prostatectomy. Seminars Radiation Oncology. 2017;**27**(1):50-66

[39] Vale CL, Fisher D, Kneebone A, et al. Adjuvant or early salvage radiotherapy for the treatment of localized and locally advanced prostate cancer: A prospectively planned systematic review and meta-analysis of aggregate data. Lancet. 2020;**396**(10260):1422-1431

[40] Valicenti RK, Thompson I Jr, Albertsen P, et al. Adjuvant and salvage

radiation therapy after prostatectomy: American Society for Radiation Oncology/American urological association guidelines. IJROBP. 2013; **86**(5):822-828

[41] Kruser TJ, Jarrard DJ, Graf AK, et al. Early hypofractionated salvage radiotherapy for prostatectomy biochemical recurrence. Cancer. 2011; **117**(12):2629-2636

[42] Katayama S, Striecker T, Kessel K, et al. Hypofractionated IMRT of the prostate bed after radical prostatectomy: Acute toxicity in the PRIAMOS-1 trial. IJROBP. 2014;**90**(4):926-933

[43] Gladwish A, Loblaw A, Cheung P, et al. Accelerated hypofractionated postoperative radiotherapy for prostate cancer: A prospective phase I/II study. Clinical Oncology (Royal College of Radiologists). 2015;**27**(3):145-152

[44] NRG-GU003: A Randomized Phase III Trial of Hypofractionated Post-Prostatectomy Radiation Therapy (HYPORT) Versus Conventional Post-Prostatectomy Radiation Therapy (COPORT). NRG Oncology. Available from: https://www.nrgoncology.org/Clinical-Trials/Protocol/nrg-gu003?filter=nrg-gu003 [Accessed: November 26, 2022]

[45] Shipley WU, Seiferheld W, Lukka H, et al. Radiation with or without antiandrogen therapy in recurrent prostate cancer. NEJM. 2017;**376**(5): 417-428

[46] Carrie C, Magné N, Burban-Provost P, et al. Short-term androgen deprivation therapy combined with radiotherapy as salvage treatment after radical prostatectomy for prostate cancer (GETUG-AFU 16): A 112-month follow-up of a phase 3, randomized trial. The Lancet Oncology. 2019;**20**(12):1740-1749

[47] Pollack A, Karrison TG, Balogh AG, et al. The addition of androgen deprivation therapy and pelvic lymph node treatment to prostate bed salvage radiotherapy (NRG oncology/RTOG 0534 SPPORT): An international, multicentre, randomized phase 3 trial. Lancet. 2022;**399**(10338):1886-1901

[48] Sheth N, Youssef I, Osborn V, et al. Association of Nadir Prostate-specific Antigen >0.5 ng/mL after dose-escalated external beam radiation with prostate cancer-specific endpoints. Cureus. 2018; **10**(6):e2790

[49] Crook J, Rodgers JP, Pisansky TM, et al. Salvage low-dose-rate prostate brachytherapy: Clinical outcomes of a phase 2 trial for local recurrence after external beam radiation therapy (NRG oncology/RTOG 0526). IJROBP. 2022; **112**(5):1115-1122

[50] Valle LF, Lehrer EJ, Markovic D, et al. A systematic review and meta-analysis of local salvage therapies after radiotherapy for prostate cancer (MASTER). European Urology. 2021; **80**(3):280-292

[51] Boevé LMS, Hulshof MCCM, Vis AN, et al. Effect on survival of androgen deprivation therapy alone compared to androgen deprivation therapy combined with concurrent radiation therapy to the prostate in patients with primary bone metastatic prostate cancer in a prospective randomised clinical trial: Data from the HORRAD trial. European Urology. 2019; **75**(3):410-418

[52] Parker CC, James ND, Brawley CD, et al. Radiotherapy to the primary tumour for newly diagnosed, metastatic prostate cancer (STAMPEDE): A randomized controlled phase 3 trial. Lancet. 2018;**392**(10162): 2353-2366

[53] Parker CC, James ND, Brawley CD, et al. Radiotherapy to the prostate for men with metastatic prostate cancer in the UK and Switzerland: Long-term results from the STAMPEDE randomized controlled trial. PLOS Medicine. 2022;**19**(6):e1003998

[54] Phillips R, Shi WY, Deek M, et al. Outcomes of observation vs stereotactic ablative radiation for Oligometastatic prostate cancer: The ORIOLE phase 2 randomized clinical trial. JAMA Oncology. 2020;**6**(5):650-659

[55] Ost P, Reynders D, Decaestecker K, et al. Surveillance or metastasis-directed therapy for Oligometastatic prostate cancer recurrence: A prospective, randomized, multicenter phase II trial. Journal of Clinical Oncology. 2018;**36**(5): 446-453

[56] Hölscher T, Baumann M, Kotzerke J, et al. Toxicity and efficacy of local ablative, image-guided radiotherapy in Gallium-68 prostate-specific membrane antigen targeted positron emission tomography-staged, castration-sensitive Oligometastatic prostate cancer: The OLI-P phase 2 clinical trial. European Urology Oncology. 2022;**5**(1):44-51

[57] Zilli T, Achard V, Dal Pra A, et al. Recommendations for radiation therapy in Oligometastatic prostate cancer: An ESTRO-ACROP Delphi consensus. Radiotherapy and Oncology. 2022;**176**: 199-207

[58] National Institutes of Health. Conventional Care Versus Radioablation (Stereotactic Body Radiotherapy) for Extracranial Oligometastases. Available from: https://clinicaltrials.gov/ct2/show /NCT02759783 [Accessed: October 14, 2022]

[59] National Institutes of Health. Management of Castration-Resistant Prostate Cancer with Oligometastases (PCS IX). Available from: https://clinicaltrials.gov/ct2/show/NCT02685397 [Accessed: October 14, 2022]

[60] National Institutes of Health. Salvage Radiotherapy Combined with Hormonotherapy in Oligometastatic Pelvic Node Relapses of Prostate Cancer (OLIGOPELVIS). Available from: https://clinicaltrials.gov/ct2/show/NCT02274779 [Accessed: October 14, 2022]

[61] National Institutes of Health. Standard Treatment +/− SBRT in Solid Tumors Patients with Between 1 and 3 Bone-Only Metastases (STEREO-OS). Available from: https://clinicaltrials.gov/ct2/show /NCT03143322 [Accessed: October 14, 2022]

[62] National Institutes of Health. PEACE V: Salvage Treatment of OligoRecurrent Nodal Prostate Cancer Metastases (STORM). Available from: https://clinicaltrials.gov/ct2/show/NCT03569241 [Accessed: October 14, 2022]

[63] Spratt DE, Zhang J, Santiago-Jiménez M, et al. Development and validation of a novel integrated clinical-genomic risk group classification for localized prostate cancer. Journal of Clinical Oncology. 2018;**36**(6):581-590

[64] Spratt DE, Huang HC, Michalski JM, et al. Validation of the performance of the decipher biopsy genomic classifier in intermediate-risk prostate cancer on the phase III randomized trial NRG oncology/RTOG 0126. Journal of Clinical Oncology. 2022;**40**(6):269

[65] Jairath NK, Dal Pra A, Vince R Jr. A systematic review of the evidence for the decipher genomic classifier in prostate cancer. European Urology. 2021;**79**(3): 374-383

[66] Lonergan PE, Washington SL, Cowan JE. Risk factors for biopsy reclassification over time in men on active surveillance for early stage prostate cancer. Journal of Urology. 2020;**204**(6):1216-1221

[67] Vince RA, Jiang R, Qi J, et al. Impact of decipher biopsy testing on clinical outcomes in localized prostate cancer in a prospective statewide collaborative. Prostate Cancer and Prostatic Diseases. 2022;**25**(4):677-683

[68] NRG Oncology. NRG-GU009. Available from: https://www.nrgoncology.org/Clinical-Trials/Protocol/nrg-gu009-1?filter=nrg-gu009-1 [Accessed: September 30, 2022]

[69] NRG Oncology. NRG-GU010. Available from: https://www.nrgoncology.org/Clinical-Trials/Protocol/nrg-gu010-1?filter=nrg-gu010-1 [Accessed: September 30, 2022]

[70] National Institutes of Health. Genomics in Michigan to AdJust Outcomes in Prostate cancer (G-MAJOR) for Men with Newly Diagnosed Favorable Risk Prostate Cancer. Available from: https://clinicaltrials.gov/ct2/show/results/NCT04396808?view=results [Accessed: September 30, 2022]

[71] Esteva A, Feng J, van der Wal D, et al. Prostate cancer therapy personalization via multi-modal deep learning on randomized phase III clinical trials. NPJ Digital Medicine. 2022;**5**(1):71

Chapter 6

SBRT in Hepatocellular Carcinoma

Carolina de la Pinta

Abstract

Stereotactic body radiation therapy (SBRT) is a precision treatment that allows high doses of radiation to be administered to the tumor volume while limiting the dose received by the surrounding healthy organs. This makes it possible to administer ablative doses to the tumor with high local control, making it an alternative in the treatment of hepatocellular carcinoma. This treatment is indicated in patients as a bridge to transplant, inoperable, or complementary treatment to other therapies such as embolization, with local control above 90% according to series. Doses and fractions are variable, and the optimal scheme has not been established. The use of this therapy has increased in recent years, although its evidence is limited. Prospective randomized studies are necessary to make this treatment the first line of action.

Keywords: SBRT, SABR, hepatocellular carcinoma, radiation therapy, radiotherapy

1. Introduction

Stereotactic body radiation therapy (SBRT) is derived from the concept of radiosurgery. The American Society of Radiation Oncology (ASTRO) describes it as high-dose, image-guided radiotherapy treatment with tumor ablative intent in a limited number of fractions. Other names used are extracranial stereotactic radiosurgery or stereotactic ablative radiotherapy (SABR) [1].

The success of radiosurgery in intracranial tumors raised interest in its application in the management of extracranial tumors. However, the development of extracranial SBRT has been much later than that of radiosurgery due to the constant internal movement of the organs by respiration and bowel movements. At the cellular level, SBRT produces cellular chromosomal damage, endothelial cell apoptosis, microvascular dysfunction, and increased lymphocyte recruitment.

ASTRO has published recommendations for SBRT treatment, and the American Association of Medical Physics Task Group 101 report has expanded on them [2, 3]. It is necessary to use systems that improve volume delineation and image fusion, including magnetic resonance and/or positron emission tomography, advanced planning algorithms, image-guided radiotherapy systems, intrafraction motion control methods, and patient immobilization systems to achieve stable and reproducible patient positioning, for which various devices that suppress or limit motion have been developed [4].

The process involves a sequence of phases, and the same applies to SBRT treatments. These phases include patient immobilization, motion assessment and management, image acquisition, image set analysis and processing, planning image fusion,

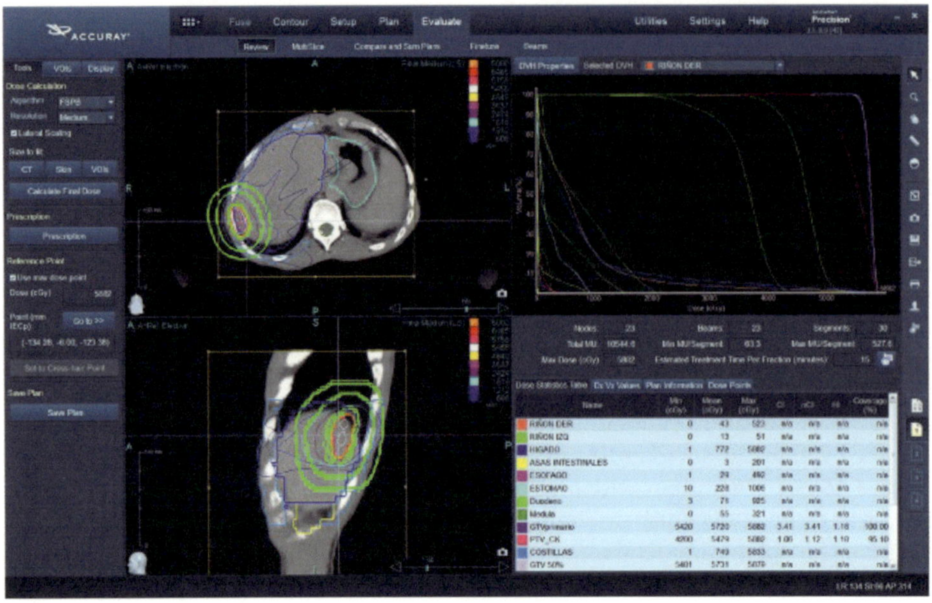

Figure 1.
Hepatocellular carcinoma planning in Cyberknife®.

volume delineation, radiation planning, quality assurance testing, patient setup in the treatment unit, acquisition of guidance images to allow target relocalization, treatment initiation, real-time monitoring of treatment integrity, and patient stability and tolerance [4].

The main obstacle that must be overcome to perform SBRT treatments involves respiratory-related motion control. Positioning errors during treatment or between treatments must also be taken into account. Image-guided radiation therapy or imaged-guided radiation therapy (IGRT) ensures target relocalization and beam alignment, which is indispensable in SBRT [4].

In SBRT, high-energy photons are used as the source of therapeutic radiation, although charged particles can also be used. There is no standard or absolute consensus solution for achieving a tightly focused high-dose distribution within the planning target volume and rapid dose fall-off outside it, the combination of beam angles or arcs best suited, and each case may present a new planning challenge. These treatments are tailored and personalized to each patient and each tumor [4]. Planning example is shown in **Figure 1**.

SBRT treatment sessions are longer than conventional treatments, so patient comfort is another important aspect, controlling patient changes in position between the time of treatment verification by imaging and treatment or even during treatment [4].

2. SBRT in hepatocellular carcinoma

2.1 Indications of SBRT in hepatocellular carcinoma (HCC)

SBRT is indicated in hepatocellular carcinoma that is not a candidate for other therapies, including surgery, radiofrequency, or transarterial chemoembolization (TACE) due to tumor location, proximity to vessels or biliary tract, and/or size. Its use in combination with the aforementioned techniques is also postulated. More evidence is needed for it to become a therapeutic modality of first choice. Data on quality of life can help in this process, making the technique not only effective, but also comfortable and with a low impact on patients' quality of life.

SBRT is an effective treatment for hepatocellular carcinoma with acceptable toxicity rates in selected patients. Despite being a procedure intended for patients who are not candidates for other treatments, it has demonstrated excellent local control in prospective and retrospective studies (studies are summarized in **Table 1**). It can be used as an exclusive treatment or in combination with other treatments. Based on the available data, it appears to complement local techniques.

The combination of SBRT and TACE offers theoretical advantages by decreasing tumor size facilitating SBRT with smaller tumors, and chemotherapy can be radiosensitizing. In addition, lipiodol is radiopaque and may aid IGRT [19].

Patients with portal vein invasion by hepatocellular carcinoma have a very poor prognosis. However, they have been included in treatment with SBRT [5–7] with encouraging results. Recanalization after SBRT facilitates treatment with TACE, which is less effective in vascular invasion. Partial and complete responses have been described with SBRT 37–75% with recanalization in 44–76% and low rates of severe toxicities [20, 21]. The maximum response time can be a few months.

Around 25–44% of patients on the transplant waiting list progress to transplantation. SBRT can help reduce this. Between 63% and 100% of patients reach transplantation with low toxicity rates and partial or complete response in 14–27% and 23–64% of lesions [22, 23]. Mohamed et al compared SBRT, TACE, radiofrequency, and Yttrium-90 microspheres as bridging therapy to transplantation in a retrospective series with 60 patients [24]. Mean necrosis was not statistically significant between treatment modalities, and toxicities were lower with SBRT and Yttrium-90. Despite being retrospective studies with few patients, it appears that SBRT is an effective and well-tolerated treatment as a bridge to transplantation and is competitive with other treatments.

Another scenario being explored is the combination with immunotherapy; the antigenic exposure produced by SBRT and the possible potentiating effect of immunotherapy, already demonstrated in other tumors, have been described. Studies are currently underway to explore the usefulness of the combined treatment of SBRT and immunotherapy due to the excellent results of immunotherapy in hepatocellular carcinoma [25].

The comparative studies available in retrospective series suggest that SBRT is a competitive treatment with other more established treatments. Given its potential, prospective comparative studies are needed [26].

2.2 Technical characteristics of SBRT in hepatocellular carcinoma

After correct immobilization of the patient, a planning CT scan is performed. The patient will be placed in supine decubitus position with the arms behind the head, avoiding that they remain in the entrance of the treatment beams. For the correct acquisition of the image, it is essential to know the contrast uptake times of each of the lesions and the need or not to use oral contrast when the stomach is close to the treatment field.

The CT image for hepatic SBRT will be acquired with intravenous contrast. The way of acquiring the contrast varies according to the location and type of tumor. The most commonly used contrast in MRI is gadolinium; however, there

Study	Child Pugh (CP)	n	Lesions	PVT (%)	Size	Doses (fr)	Follow-up	OS (2 a)	Toxicity
Lasley et al Phase-I-II (2015) [5]	A B7/8+: 81/19	59	39 26	20	33.6 cc (2.0–107.3)	48Gy (36–48)/3) CPB: 40/5 Median 30Gy (6)	33.3 m CP A 46.3 m CP B	2-y: 72% CPA 33% CPB 3-y: 61% CPA 26% CPB	Liver: 4 p CPA 8p CPB Grade 3/4
Kang et al Phase-II (2012) [6]	A B/AC	41 6 5	56	11	2.9cc (1.3–7.8)	42–60Gy (3)	17 m	68.7%	Gastrointestial:3p Grade 3 2p Grade 4
Culleton et al (2014) [7]	B7/8/9: 69/24/3 C10:3	29		76		30Gy (6)		1-y 32%	63% had decline in CP score by 2 or more at 3 months
Méndez Romero et al phase II (2006) [8]			45 11 HCC	25	3.5cc (0.5–7.2)	25Gy (5) 30Gy (3)	12.9 m	1-y 75%	4p =>Grade 3 1p CP B liver failure
Sanuki et al (2014) [9]	A B/A	137 48	185	—	<5cm	40Gy 35Gy	24 m	3-y: 70%	24p >Grade 3 19 p worse 2 points CP 2p G5 liver failure
Su et al (2016) [10]	A B/AC	114 18	175	—	3cm (1.1–5.0)	42–46 Gy (3–5) 28–30Gy (1)	21 m	1-y: 94.1% 3-y: 73.5% 5-y: 64.3%	11p => Grade 3
Scorsetti et al (2015) [11]	A B	43	63	20	4.8cc (1–12.5)	48–75Gy (3) 36–60Gy (6)	8 m	1-y: 77.9+/−8.2 2-y: 43.5+/−14	7p =>Grade 3 No RILD
Bujold et al Phase-I-II (2013) [12]	A/ AC	102 55		55	7.2cc (1.4–23.1)	36 (24–54)/6	31.4 m	1 a: 55%	=> Grade 3 30%
Yamashita et al (2015) [13]	A B	67 9		—		48 Gy (4) (40Gy/4– 60Gy/10)	21 m	2-y: 53%	No Grade 3

DOI: http://dx.doi.org/10.5772/intechopen.109622

Study	Child Pugh (CP)	n	Lesions	PVT (%)	Size	Doses (fr)	Follow-up	OS (2 a)	Toxicity
Andolino et al (2011) [14]	A B /AC	36 24	60		3.2 cm	44Gy (3) 40Gy (8)	27 m	67%	No =>Grade 3 13% liver >Grade 1 20% worse CP
Bibault et al (2013) [15]	A B/AC	67 8	96	—	3.7cm (3.0–4.4)	40–45 (3)	10 m	1-y: 78.5% 2-y: 50.4%	No => Grade 3
Park et al (2013) [16]		26	28		<6cm	40–50Gy (10)		1-y: 88.5% 2-y: 67.2%	>Grade 3 1 p
Takeda et al (2014) [17]		73		—		35–40Gy (5)	31.3 m	1-y: 100% 2-y: 87% 3-y: 73%	Liver Grade 3 = 32 p
Wahl et al (2016) [18]	A B C	57 24 2	83	—	2.2 cm	30–50Gy		1-y: 70% 2-y: 53%	Grade >3 3p

HCC: hepatocellular carcinoma, PVT: portal vein thrombosis, OS: overall survival, and RILD: radio-induced liver disease.

Table 1.
Retrospective and prospective studies of hepatocellular carcinoma SBRT.

are organ-specific contrasts in MRI, and these are mainly used in the diagnosis of focal hepatic lesions in which previous imaging tests have been inconclusive. The three agents that have been developed for this purpose are mangafodipir trisodium (Mn-DPDP), gadobenate dimeglumine (Gd-BOPTA), and gadoxetic acid (Gd-EOB-DTPA). Poorly differentiated HCC does not pick up these contrasts, but it has been described that some well-differentiated hepatocellular carcinoma may do so.

2.2.1 Image acquisition in hepatocellular carcinoma

Because of its special behavior, CT contrast acquisition for hepatocellular carcinoma is somewhat different from other tumors. In the normal liver, hepatic irrigation is mainly by the portal vein and to a lesser extent by the hepatic artery. In the process of hepatocarcinogenesis, arterial vascularization predominates over portal vascularization. For this reason, the diagnosis of hepatocellular carcinoma is based on its vascular behavior and radiological studies are performed with contrast in arterial, portal, and late phases, in addition to alpha-fetoprotein levels and histological analysis.

The typical radiological characteristics of hepatocellular carcinoma in both CT and MRI in the dynamic study are contrast hyperenhancement in the arterial phase with early washout in the late phase, the latter phase being decisive for the diagnosis as it becomes hypodense/hypointense with respect to the normal liver parenchyma, presenting in some cases a pseudocapsule image. Another important characteristic of hepatocellular carcinoma is its internal mosaic appearance due to the presence of areas with different density in CT or heterogeneous signal in MRI that mainly appear in the postcontrast study.

Sometimes hepatocellular carcinoma can be hypovascular and show no arterial hypervascularization, in which case the portal and late phases are very important, where they remain hypodense/hypointense or even have atypical behavior with hyperenhancement in the arterial phase and absence of late washout [27].

The signal characteristics of hepatocellular carcinoma on MRI is variable. In T1-weighted sequences, about one-third are seen as hypointense lesions, one-third are isointense, and another third are hyperintense (due to hemorrhage or fatty degeneration). In T2-weighted sequences, the signal intensity is closely related to the degree of malignancy, and the higher the degree of malignancy the more hyperintense in T2. Sometimes, there may be hypointense areas in T2 sequences, related to the presence of a scar, old bleeding (hemosiderin), or necrosis. In cases in which the capsule is present, it is hypointense in T1 and hyperintense in the postcontrast study. Fat deposition is easy to demonstrate on MRI (up to 14%) using T1 sequences. Peritumoral edema corresponding to compressed liver parenchyma can be seen in approximately 20% of cases. In diffusion sequences, hepatocellular carcinoma shows signal hyperintensity, with low ADC values, which translates a diffusion restriction due to high cellularity.

2.2.2 Volume delineation

The imaging test used in the calculation algorithms for radiotherapy is CT; however, the definition of the gross tumor volume (GTV) in planning CT in liver tumors sometimes requires the use of supporting imaging tests that allow a correct visualization of the tumor, including different phases, sequences, or contrast acquisition times.

The efficacy of SBRT is totally dependent on the delimitation of the GTV, and an erroneous delimitation would mean on the one hand leaving tumor volume out of the irradiation field and on the other hand irradiating more healthy tissue than necessary, increasing the possibility of side effects.

The definition of the GTV in hepatocellular carcinoma requires the identification of abnormal areas in all phases of a multiphase CT and/or MRI. The definition of GTV typically represents a union of these findings. When vascular thrombosis is present, the definition of the lesion is more complex and is best visualized in the venous or late phases, requiring multiple images [28]. In liver metastases and pancreatic adenocarcinoma, PET/CT could be of added value in tumor delimitation to CT and/or MRI, although it is difficult to define the borderline uptake area (SUV).

2.3 Local control with SBRT in hepatocellular carcinoma

In the literature, there are multiple prospective studies, phase I and II, of SBRT in hepatocellular carcinoma with local control at 2 years ranging from 64 to 95% (**Table 1**).

Méndez Romero et al published the first prospective study in 2006. Eight patients had hepatocellular carcinoma with 11 lesions larger than 7 cm. Dose prescription was based on lesion size and the presence of cirrhosis. Local control at 1 year was 75%. Local failure was only observed at low doses (25 Gy in 5 fractions) [8]. Kang et al published a phase II study including patients with incomplete response to TACE and Child Pugh A. Local control at 2 years after SBRT (42–60Gy in three fractions) was 95% [6].

Two of the retrospective studies with the largest number of patients are the study by Sanuki et al, in 2013, and Su et al [9, 10]. The former included 185 patients with 185 lesions, <=5cm. The prescription doses were 40 and 35 Gy for Child Pugh A and B, respectively, in five fractions. Local control at 3 years was 91%19. In the study by Su et al, the authors who published the result of 114 Child Pugh A and 18 B non-candidates for other treatments, with 175 lesions, all less than or equal to 5 cm treated with 42–46 Gy in 3–5 fractions, local control at 1 year was 91% [10].

Recently, Rim et al performed a systematic review and meta-analysis analyzing 32 studies with 1950 patients, including local control and overall survival (OS) as the primary objective, and toxicity as a secondary objective. Local control at 3 years was 83.9%. The median tumor size was 3.3 cm (1.6–8.6 cm). The median dose, calculated in EQD2 (equivalent dose in 2 Gy fractions), was 48–114.8Gy (median 83.3 Gy). Concluding that SBRT in hepatocellular carcinoma provides excellent local control at 3 years [29]. Most of these studies include patients with hepatocellular carcinoma in Child Pugh A and B cirrhotic livers. In all of them, there is great heterogeneity in dosimetric parameters with doses ranging from 12 Gy in three fractions to 55 Gy in five fractions.

2.4 Treatment schedules with SBRT in hepatocellular carcinoma: Dose and fractionation

A wide variety of doses and fractions have been described for the treatment of hepatocellular carcinoma with SBRT. These doses vary according to different studies from 30 to 50 Gy in 3–6 fractions. Liver function and the dose received by healthy organs influence the choice of the prescription dose. Some studies have shown that the administration of higher doses is decisive for local control and overall survival, but others have not. In fact, hepatocellular carcinoma is considered a radiosensitive tumor, such that, above a threshold dose, there may be little benefit in additional doses with increased toxicity. For small tumors far from healthy tissues (especially gastrointestinal organs), 40 Gy in five fractions can be used. For larger tumors, where doses must be limited due to hepatic tolerance, individualized schedules can be used in each prescription [11, 30]. In addition, this may vary according to the treatment planning technique.

Prescribing doses have not yet been fully defined; there are many different treatment schedules in the literature. It is important to emphasize that patients with Child Pugh stages B 8–9 and C are underrepresented in SBRT studies [29, 31]. When they are included, radiotherapy doses are reduced. Given the underrepresentation of these patients in studies, Culleton et al published prospective (14 patients) and retrospective (15 patients) data with Child Pugh B and C, 76% with portal vein tumor invasion and 24% with extrahepatic disease. The median dose prescribed was 30 Gy in six fractions. Overall survival was 32% at 1 year and better in patients with Child Pugh B7 compared to higher Child Pugh. Progression at 1 year was 45%, and worsening of functional class 2 was observed in 63% at 3 months. The most common side effect was Grade 1–2 asthenia. There were no toxicities greater than or equal to grade 3. There was no tumor progression despite lowering the dose. Sixty percent of patients died in the first year due to liver disease with or without active hepatocellular carcinoma. Elevated AFP was associated with worse survival [7]. Dose recommendations have recently been published by the ASTRO [26].

2.5 Side effects with SBRT in hepatocellular carcinoma

In addition to the doses in the treatment volume, the assessment of doses in healthy organs, in the unaffected liver, and in gastrointestinal organs is very important.

Radio-induced liver toxicity, radio-induced hepatitis, or radio-induced liver disease (RILD) is a form of subacute liver damage due to radiotherapeutic treatment. However, it has been described in other treatments such as chemotherapy administration and in conditioning for marrow transplantation. It is one of the most feared complications in radiotherapeutic treatment and hinders dose escalation and re-irradiation of hepatobiliary or lower gastrointestinal tract tumors [32, 33].

Biliary toxicity includes the risk of biliary stricture, duodenal, gastric or intestinal toxicity, ulceration, and perforation. ASTRO has recently published tolerance recommendations for these organs at risk [28]; see **Table 2**.

Other studies include dose limits in large vessels and esophagus. Tolerance limits in large vessels include doses of 50Gy/5 fractions (40–60Gy, 3–5 fractions) and maximum dose on large vessels of 52.5Gy in five fractions with a grade 3 toxicity of 0.2%, grade 4 of 0%, and grade 5 of 0.3%26. Esophageal dose limits include maximum doses of 32.3–43.4 Gy in five fractions or 35Gy in four fractions [34].

2.6 Factors of response in SBRT of hepatocellular carcinoma

2.6.1 Local control

In the literature, there is great heterogeneity of doses, and the optimal dose has not been established. The aim is to develop models of the dose-control relationship in order to optimize treatment. Lausch et al used their data to develop a model, including 36 patients with hepatocellular carcinoma treated with a median of 4 Gy in each session (2–10 Gy), with a total median dose of 52 Gy (29–83 Gy). The investigators demonstrated radiosensitivity of hepatocellular carcinoma with respect to liver

Organ at risk	Three fractions	five fractions	Toxicity
Liver, non-cirrhosis	Median < 12–15Gy > 700cc>19Gy	Median < 15–18Gy > 700cc <21Gy	RILD
Liver, CP A	Media < 10–12Gy	Median < 13–15Gy >700cc<15Gy	Increase in CP > 2 at 3 months
Liver, CP B7	—	Median < 8–10 Gy >500cc < 10Gy	Increase in CP > 2 at 3 months RILD
Biliary tract	D0.03cc < 37.7Gy	D0.03cc > 40.5Gy	Stenosis
Gastric	D0.03cc < 22Gy D10cc < 16.5Gy	D0.03cc < 32Gy D10cc < 18Gy	Ulcer
Duodenum	D0.03cc < 22Gy D5cc < 16.5Gy	D0.03cc < 32Gy D5cc < 18Gy	Ulcer
Small bowel	D0.03cc < 25Gy D5cc < 18Gy	D0.03cc < 32Gy D5cc < 19.5Gy	Ulcer
Large bowel	D0.03cc < 28Gy D5cc < 24Gy	D0.03cc < 34Gy D5cc < 25Gy	Ulcer

Table 2.
Dose-limiting organ risk dose recommendations for liver and luminal structures according to ASTRO guideline [26].

metastases, including colorectal metastases, and suggested that increasing the dose increases local control [35]. Jang et al developed a model based on tumor size, demonstrating that high doses are necessary to achieve tumor control in large lesions [12]. In addition, a Tumor Control Probability (TCP) model has recently been published with multi-institutional data, including a total of 431 patients with hepatocellular carcinoma, concluding that there does not appear to be a dose-response relationship in SBRT in hepatocellular carcinoma. The authors recommend conservative schedules in hepatocellular carcinoma, such as 8–10 Gy per fraction in five fractions; doses >50 Gy in five fractions increase the risk of toxicity without improving local control [36]. In the study by Cardenes et al, dose escalation from 36 Gy, with increments of 2 Gy in 2 Gy, was studied, finding that the dose of 48 Gy in three fractions (Biological Effective Dose (BED) = 125 Gy, EQD2 EQD2 =104 Gy) presented a local control at 2 years of 90% and minimal toxicity [37]. Jang et al found that an increase in EQD2 from 104Gy to 126Gy resulted in an increase in local control from 90 to 100% [30]. Yamashita et al analyzed the treatment of 79 patients with hepatocellular carcinoma, finding no difference in local control with doses above and below 100 Gy of biologic equivalent dose. Their local control at 2 years was statistically different when comparing lesions above and below 3 cm in maximum diameter (local control 64% vs. 85%) [13]. The dose response may simply reflect the variation in lesion size in different trials and the ability to give a high dose in small lesions.

2.6.2 Overall survival

Another major topic of discussion is whether dose is related to survival. In 2013, a prospective study with 102 patients with Child Pugh A hepatocellular carcinoma, Bujold et al demonstrated that patients receiving <30 Gy in six fractions (BED=45 Gy, EQD2=38 Gy) vs. 30 Gy had local control at 2 years 66% vs. 85% [12]. This difference did not translate into improved overall survival, being, however, the major cause of progression. These data suggest that dose escalation does not increase overall survival. A Korean study by Seong et al included 398 patients (Child Pugh A 73.9%) from 10 different centers. This study demonstrated an overall survival benefit for patients who received BED>=53Gy [38]. Dose escalation is limited by the tolerance of the organs at risk. There are nomograms and multivariate models that demonstrate that liver function, especially in Child Pugh B and C, and tumor size are more determinant in survival compared to dose escalation. Although dose correlates with local control, and local control with overall survival, only in a minority of patients does it result in a survival benefit. Doses in hepatocellular carcinoma higher than 84 Gy do not seem to be justified by the minimal increase in local control and significant increase in toxicity. In the study by Myungsoo et al, a tumor volume greater or less than 214 cm^3 and a total dose greater or less than 105 Gy of effective biological dose were established as prognostic factors for progression-free survival. Based on these factors, patients were divided into a favorable and unfavorable prognostic group. Local progression-free survival and overall survival were better in the favorable group than in the unfavorable group (2-year local progression-free survival rate: 51.3% vs. 30.0%, 2-year OS rate: 72.8% vs. 30.0%) [39].

3. Overall survival

Overall survival is around 66.7% at 3 years [40]. In the study by Méndez Romero et al, overall survival at 1 year was 75%18 and in the study by Bujold et al, 55% (24–54 Gy in six fractions) [12]. And in the study by Su et al, overall survival at 1 year was 94%20. Kang et al reported an OS at 2 years after SBRT (42–60 Gy in three fractions) of 69% [6]. In the study by Sanuki et al, overall survival at 3 years was 70%, with no difference between doses of 35 and 40 Gy [9]. Overall survival at 1, 2, and 3 years in the study by Rim et al. was 72.6, 57.8, and 48.3%, respectively [29].

When the intention of the treatment is neoadjuvant, the aim is to prevent progression of patients on the waiting list for liver transplantation and to prevent them from leaving the waiting list. SBRT is an effective treatment as a bridge to transplantation. One study retrospectively included 10 patients with hepatocellular carcinoma on the transplant list treated with SBRT. Two patients had Child Pugh B and one had Child Pugh C, the median tumor size was 3.4 cm (2.5–5.5 cm), and the median dose was 51 Gy in 3 fractions. Four patients had received previous treatment with TACE. All patients were successfully transplanted. On anatomic-pathologic review, three patients had complete response and three patients had minimal remainder. The 5-year overall survival and progression-free survival were 100%, and there were no toxicities greater than or equal to grade 3 [41]. Mannina et al analyzed their experience using SBRT in 38 patients with hepatocellular carcinoma, and all patients were transplanted [40]. Complete response was observed in 45% of lesions and partial response in 23%, with poor concordance between radiological and pathological evaluation. Overall survival at 1, 2, 3, and 5 years was 92, 86, 77, and 73%, respectively [42].

4. Evaluation of response

The Response Evaluation Criteria In Solid Tumors (RECIST) v1.1 criteria take into account changes in tumor size, underestimating the detection of complete response and overestimating partial responses. Disappearance of arterial hyperenhancement is considered a complete response, while a 30% reduction is a partial response and a 20% increase is progression [43, 44]. If none of these changes is present, it is considered stable disease. Different criteria may be useful for ablation, embolization, or systemic treatment, but their application in SBRT is unclear. Most clinical trials of SBRT in hepatocellular carcinoma use these criteria for response assessment, and there is a need to standardize the response by unifying the imaging changes observed after SBRT in hepatocellular carcinoma. Facciuto et al showed correlation of RECIST v1.1 with complete response in 14% of patients at 3 months [23]. Mannina et al retrospectively evaluated 38 patients with hepatocellular carcinoma (Child Pugh A 45%) treated with SBRT prior to transplantation and demonstrated low concordance of complete responses or partial response with RECIST (sensitivity 90% and specificity 17%), mRECIST (sensitivity 54% and specificity 50%), and European Association for the Study of the Liver (EASL) (sensitivity 83% and specificity 18%); however, no patient was incorrectly categorized to progression [42].

The timing of imaging response assessment is crucial. Sanuki et al demonstrated median time to complete response of 5.9 months (1.2–34.2 months) [45]. Complete response increased from 24% at 3 months to 67% at 6 months and 71% at 12 months. Kimura et al demonstrated that 25.3% had residual arterial hyperenhancement at 3 months, which decreased significantly to 2% at 6 months [46]. Price et al demonstrated discordance between response assessment by EASL and RECIST [47]. Evaluating the mean decrease in tumor size (RECIST), they found 35, 37, 48, and 55% reduction at 3, 6, 9, and 12 months, respectively. However, a decrease in arterial enhancement of 50% (partial response by EASL) was more predictive of response in the first 6 to 12 months.

After SBRT, there are changes in the surrounding liver tissue. According to these changes, some authors have described temporal changes in hyperenhancement, corresponding to areas of high dose, finding an increase in hyperenhancement from 12% at 1 month to 54% at 6 months. The delay in image acquisition shows isoattenuation in most patients, being rare in the late phase, which may help to distinguish the response to treatment. In addition, the degree of cirrhosis may predict different behavior [45]. Kimura et al found that the majority of tumors in Child Pugh A patients went from hypo- or isoattenuation to hyperattenuation within 6 months of treatment; however, no such changes were seen in Child Pugh B patients. It should be noted that the optimal response time is at least 6 to 12 months after SBRT, lesion stability, or shrinkage is associated with local treatment success, arterial phase hyperenhancement may persist despite complete pathologic response, and late washout may persist after SBRT [48]. Some of these lesions may be incorrectly categorized as treatment failures by administering unnecessary additional treatments.

5. Quality of life with SBRT in hepatocellular carcinoma

The available evidence is limited, and the assessment tools vary from study to study. There are no studies limited to the evaluation of quality of life in patients with primary and secondary liver tumors. Moreover, there are differences in these pathologies that make it difficult to group them together. However, the change in quality of life in oncology patients after treatment can be substantial.

A systematic review published by Mutsaers et al [49] evaluated the quality of life of patients after treatment with SBRT in primaries or liver metastases. A total of 392 patients from four prospective studies and one abstract were analyzed. The review concludes that quality of life is preserved after SBRT treatment.

The prospective longitudinal study by Klein et al [50] using the FACT-Hep and QLQ-C30 quality of life questionnaires included 99 patients with hepatocellular carcinoma. Loss of appetite and asthenia worsened at 1 month, but recovered by 3 months, with no significant changes in quality of life in the series. Shun et al [51] found factors, including depression, functional status, and symptom severity associated with changes in quality of life. Nutritional status and mental health during treatment could affect quality of life. The most common changes were asthenia and nutritional status.

There is little evidence to compare quality of life data from SBRT with other treatments such as radiofrequency, TACE, or surgery. If we review quality of life after other local treatments, the studies by Rees et al [52] (liver resection) and Toro et al [53] (liver resection, TACE, radiofrequency, or no treatment) suggest a stable score; however, the studies by Eid et al [54] (liver resection or ablation) and Huang et al [55] (resection vs. radiofrequency) suggest a worsening. Similar variations are seen post-chemo/Yttrium-90 [56]. Based on this limited data analysis, SBRT is a comparable or favorable alternative to other techniques.

6. Conclusion

SBRT treatment of hepatocellular carcinoma is an effective treatment with limited complications. More studies are needed to establish definitive indications, response and survival factors, and evaluation of response to treatment.

Acknowledgements

I would like to thank Hospital Ramón y Cajal and the research foundation of Hospital Ramón y Cajal for their support.

Conflict of interest

The authors declare no conflict of interest.

Author details

Carolina de la Pinta
Ramón y Cajal Hospital, IRYCIS, Madrid, Spain

*Address all correspondence to: cdelapintaa@gmail.com

References

[1] Gunderson and Tepper. Clinical Radiation Oncology. 4th ed. Philadelphia: Elsevier; 2016

[2] Potters L, Kavanagh B, Galvin JM, et al. American society for therapeutic radiology and oncology (ASTRO) and American college of radiology (ACR) practice guideline for the performance of stereotactic body radiation therapy. International Journal of Radiation Oncology, Biology, Physics. 2010;**76**(2):326-332

[3] Benedict SH, Yenice KM, Followill D, et al. Stereotactic body radiation therapy: The report of AAPM task group 101. Medical Physics. 2010;**37**(8):4078-4101

[4] Fernández-Letón P, Baños C, Bea J, Delgado Rodríguez JM, De Blas PR, Martínez Ortega J, et al. Recomendaciones de la Sociedad Española de Física Médica (SEFM) sobre implementación y uso clínico de radioterapia estereotáxica extracraneal (SBRT). SEFM Revised Fisihery Medical. 2017;**18**(2):1-11

[5] Lasley FD, Mannina EM, Johnson CS. Treatment variables related to liver toxicity in patients with hepatocellular carcinoma, Child-Pugh class A and B enrolled in a phase 1-2 trial of stereotactic body radiation therapy. Practical Radiation Oncology. 2015;**5**(5):e443-e449

[6] Kang JK, Kim MS, Cho CK. Stereotactic body radiation therapy for inoperable hepatocellular carcinoma as a local salvage treatment after incomplete transarterial chemoembolization. Cancer. 2012;**118**(21):5424-5431

[7] Culleton S, Jiang H, Haddad CR. Outcomes following definitive stereotactic body radiotherapy for patients with Child-Pugh B or C hepatocellular carcinoma. Radiotherapy and Oncology. 2014;**111**(3):412-417

[8] Méndez Romero A, Wunderink W, Hussain SM, De Pooter JA, Heijmen BJ, Nowak PC, et al. Stereotactic body radiation therapy for primary and metastatic liver tumors: A single institution phase I-II study. Acta Oncologica. 2006;**45**(7):831-837. DOI: 10.1080/02841860600897934

[9] Sanuki N, Takeda A, Oku Y. Stereotactic body radiotherapy for small hepatocellular carcinoma: A retrospective outcome analysis in 185 patients. Acta Oncologica. 2014;**53**(3):399-404

[10] Su TS, Liang P, Lu HZ. Stereotactic body radiation therapy for small primary or recurrent hepatocellular carcinoma in 132 Chinese patients. Journal of Surgical Oncology. 2016;**113**(2):181-187

[11] Scorsetti M, Comito T, Cozzi L. The challenge of inoperable hepatocellular carcinoma (HCC): Results of a single-institutional experience on stereotactic body radiation therapy (SBRT). Journal of Cancer Research and Clinical Oncology. 2015;**141**(7):1301-1309

[12] Bujold A, Massey CA, Kim JJ. Sequential phase I and II trials of stereotactic body radiotherapy for locally advanced hepatocellular carcinoma. Journal of Clinical Oncology. 2013;**31**(13):1631-1639

[13] Yamashita H, Onishi H, Murakami N, et al. Survival outcomes after stereotactic body radiotherapy for 79 Japanese patients with hepatocellular carcinoma. Journal of Radiation Research. 2015;**56**:561-567

[14] Andolino DL, Johnson CS, Maluccio M, Kwo P, Tector AJ, Zook J, et al. Stereotactic body radiotherapy for primary hepatocellular carcinoma. International Journal of Radiation Oncology, Biology, Physics. 2011;**81**(4):e447-e453. DOI: 10.1016/j.ijrobp.2011.04.011

[15] Bibault JE, Dewas S, Vautravers-Dewas C, Hollebecque A, Jarraya H, Lacornerie T, et al. Stereotactic body radiation therapy for hepatocellular carcinoma: Prognostic factors of local control, overall survival, and toxicity. PLoS One. 2013;**8**(10):e77472. DOI: 10.1371/journal.pone.0077472

[16] Park JH, Yoon SM, Lim YS, Kim SY, Shim JH, Kim KM, et al. Two-week schedule of hypofractionated radiotherapy as a local salvage treatment for small hepatocellular carcinoma. Journal of Gastroenterology and Hepatology. 2013;**28**(10):1638-1642. DOI: 10.1111/jgh.12249

[17] Takeda A, Sanuki N, Eriguchi T, Kobayashi T, Iwabutchi S, Matsunaga K, et al. Stereotactic ablative body radiotherapy for previously untreated solitary hepatocellular carcinoma. Journal of Gastroenterology and Hepatology. 2014;**29**(2):372-379. DOI: 10.1111/jgh.12350

[18] Wahl DR, Stenmark MH, Tao Y, Pollom EL, Caoili EM, Lawrence TS, et al. Outcomes After Stereotactic Body Radiotherapy or Radiofrequency Ablation for Hepatocellular Carcinoma. Journal of Clinical Oncology. 2016;**34**(5):452-459. DOI: 10.1200/JCO.2015.61.4925

[19] Zhao J, Zeng L, Wu Q, Wang L, Lei J, Luo H, et al. Stereotactic body radiotherapy combined with transcatheter arterial chemoembolization versus stereotactic body radiotherapy alone as the first-line treatment for unresectable hepatocellular carcinoma: A meta-analysis and systematic review. Chemotherapy. 2019;**64**(5-6):248-258. DOI: 10.1159/000505739

[20] Xi M, Zhang L, Zhao L. Effectiveness of stereotactic body radiotherapy for hepatocellular carcinoma with portal vein and/or inferior vena cava tumor thrombosis. PLoS One. 2013;**8**(5):e63864

[21] Choi BO, Choi IB, Jang HS. Stereotactic body radiation therapy with or without transarterial chemoembolization for patients with primary hepatocellular carcinoma: Preliminary analysis. BMC Cancer. 2008;**8**:351

[22] Barry AS, Sapisichin G, Russo M. The use of stereotactic body radiotherapy as a bridge to liver transplantation for hepatocellular carcinoma. Journal of Clinical Oncology. 2016;**34**(suppl 1 and 4):S1

[23] Facciuto ME, Singh MK, Rochon C. Stereotactic body radiation therapy in hepatocellular carcinoma and cirrhosis: Evaluation of radiological and pathological response. Journal of Surgical Oncology. 2012;**105**(7):692-698

[24] Mohamed M, Katz AW, Tejani MA. Comparison of outcomes between SBRT, yttrium-90 radioembolization, transarterial chemoembolization, and radiofrequency ablation as bridge to transplant for hepatocellular carcinoma. Advances in Radiation Oncology. 2016;**1**:8

[25] Kreidieh M, Zeidan YH, Shamseddine A. The Combination of Stereotactic Body Radiation Therapy and Immunotherapy in Primary Liver Tumors. Journal of Oncology. 2019;**2019**:4304817. DOI: 10.1155/2019/4304817

[26] Apisarnthanarax S, Barry A, Cao M, Czito B, DeMatteo R, Drinane M, et al. External beam radiation therapy for primary liver cancers: An ASTRO Clinical Practice Guideline. Practical Radiation Oncology. 2021;**S1879**(21):00233. DOI: 10.1016/j.prro.2021.09.004

[27] Castaño Palacio DM, Caba Cuevas M, Cigüenza Sancho M, Tejerina A, González Ortega S, del Campo del Val L. Diagnóstico por imagen del Hepatocarcinoma (HCC): hallazgos típicos y atípicos en tomografía computerizada (TC) y resonancia magnética (RM). Utilidad de los contrastes órgano-específicos. SERAM. 2012;**2012**:S-1149. DOI: 10.1594/seram2012/S-1149

[28] Hong TS, Bosch WR, Krishnan S, Kim TK, Mamon HJ, Shyn P, et al. Interobserver variability in target definition for hepatocellular carcinoma with and without portal vein thrombus: Radiation Therapy Oncology Group Consensus Guidelines. International Journal of Radiation Oncology, Biology, Physics. 2014;**89**(4):804-813

[29] Rim CH, Kim HJ, Seong J. Clinical feasibility and efficacy of stereotactic body radiotherapy for hepatocellular carcinoma: A systematic review and meta-analysis of observational studies. Radiotherapy Oncology. 2019;**131**:135-144

[30] Jang WI, Kim MS, Bae SH. High-dose stereotactic body radiotherapy correlates increased local control and overall survival in patients with inoperable hepatocellular carcinoma. Radiation Oncology. 2013;**8**:250

[31] Jang WI, Bae SH, Kim MS, Han CJ, Park SC, Kim SB, et al. A phase 2 multicenter study of stereotactic body radiotherapy for hepatocellular carcinoma: Safety and efficacy. Cancer. 2020;**126**(2):363-372. DOI: 10.1002/cncr.32502

[32] De La Pinta Alonso C. Radiation-induced liver disease in the era of SBRT: A review. Expert Review of Gastroenterology & Hepatology. 2020 Dec;**14**(12):1195-1201. DOI: 10.1080/17474124.2020.1814744

[33] Xue J, Kubicek G, Patel A, et al. Validity of current stereotactic body radiation therapy dose constraints for aorta and major vessels. Seminatic Radiation Oncology. 2016;**26**:135-139

[34] Nuyttens JJ, Moiseenko V, McLaughlin M, et al. Esophageal dose tolerance in patients treated with stereotactic body radiation therapy. Seminars in Radiation Oncology. 2016;**26**:120-128

[35] Lausch A, Sinclair K, Lock M, et al. Determination and comparison of radiotherapy dose responses for hepatocellular carcinoma and metastatic colorectal liver tumours. The British Journal of Radiology. 2013;**86**(1027):20130147

[36] Ohri N, Tomé WA, Méndez Romero A, Miften M, Ten Haken RK, Dawson LA, et al. Local control after stereotactic body radiation therapy for liver tumors. International Journal of Radiation Oncology, Biology, Physics. 2021;**110**(1):188-195. DOI: 10.1016/j.ijrobp.2017.12.288

[37] Cardenes HR, Price TR, Perkins SM, et al. Phase I feasibility trial of stereotactic body radiation therapy for primary hepatocellular carcinoma. Clinical Translational Oncology. 2010;**12**(3):218-225

[38] Seong J, Lee IJ, Shim SJ, et al. A multicenter retrospective cohort study of practice patterns and clinical outcome

on radiotherapy for hepatocellular carcinoma in Korea. Liver International. 2009;**29**(2):147-152

[39] Kim M, Seung Kay C, Won J, et al. Prognostic value of tumor volumen and radiation dose in moderate-sized hepatocellular carcinoma. A multicenter analysis in Korea (KROG 14-17). Medicine. 2017;**96**:er202

[40] Weiner AA, Olsen J, Ma D, et al. Stereotactic body radiotherapy for primary hepatic malignancies—report of a phase I/II institutional study. Radiotherapy and Oncology. 2016;**121**:79-85

[41] Sapisochin G, Barry A, Doherty M, et al. Grant DR: Stereotactic body radiotherapy vs TACE or RFA as a bridge to transplant in patients with hepatocellular carcinoma: An intention-to-treat analysis. Journal of Hepatology. 2017;**67**:92-99

[42] Mannina EM, Cardenes HR, Lasley FD, et al. Role of stereotactic body radiation therapy before orthotopic liver transplantation: Retrospective evaluation of pathologic response and outcomes. International Journal of Radiation Oncology, Biology, Physics. 2017;**97**:931-938

[43] Lencioni R, Llovet JM. Modified RECIST (mRECIST) assessment for hepatocellular carcinoma. Seminars in Liver Disease. 2010;**30**(1):52-60

[44] Vincenzi B, Di Maio M, Silletta M, et al. Prognostic relevance of objective response according to EASL criteria and mRECIST criteria in hepatocellular carcinoma patients treated with loco-regional therapies: A literature-based meta-analysis. PLoS One. 2015;**10**(7):e0133488

[45] Sanuki N, Takeda A, Mizuno T, et al. Tumor response on CT following hypofractionated stereotactic ablative body radiotherapy for small hypervascular hepatocellular carcinoma with cirrhosis. AJR. American Journal of Roentgenology. 2013;**201**(6):W812-W820

[46] Kimura T, Takahashi S, Kenjo M, et al. Dynamic computed tomography appearance of tumor response after stereotactic body radiation therapy for hepatocellular carcinoma: How should we evaluate treatment effects? Hepatology Research. 2013;**43**(7):717-727

[47] Price TR, Perkins SM, Sandrasegaran K, et al. Evaluation of response after stereotactic body radiotherapy for hepatocellular carcinoma. Cancer. 2012;**118**(12):3191-3198

[48] Mendiratta-Lala M, Gu E, Owen D, et al. Imaging findings within the first 12 months of hepatocellular carcinoma treated with stereotactic body radiation therapy. International Journal of Radiation Oncology, Biology, Physics. 2018;**2017**

[49] Mutsaers A, Greenspoon J, Walker-Dilks C, et al. Systematic review of patient reported quality of life following stereotactic ablative radiotherapy for primary and metastatic liver cancer. Radiation Oncology. 2017;**12**(1):110

[50] Klein J, Dawson LA, Jiang H, et al. Prospective longitudinal assessment of quality of life for liver cancer patients treated with stereotactic body radiation therapy. International Journal of Radiational Oncology Biology. 2015;**93**:16-25

[51] Shun S, Chiou J, Lai Y, Yu P, et al. Changes in quality of life and its related factors in liver cancer patients receiving stereotactic radiation therapy. Supportive Care in Cancer. 2008;**16**:1059-1065

[52] Rees J, Blazeby J, Brookes S, John T, Welsh F, Rees M. Patient-reported outcomes in long-term survivors of metastatic colorectal cancer needing liver resection. The British Journal of Surgery. 2014;**101**:1468-1474

[53] Toro A, Pulvirenti E, Palermo F, Di Carlo I. Health-related quality of life in patients with hepatocellular carcinoma after hepatic resection, transcatheter arterial chemoembolization, radiofrequency ablation or no treatment. Surgical Oncology. 2012;**21**:e23-e30

[54] Eid S, Stromberg A, Ames S, Ellis S, McMasters K, Martin R. Assessment of symptom experience in patients undergoing hepatic resection or ablation. Cancer. 2006;**107**:2715-2722

[55] Huang G, Chen X, Lau W, Shen F, Wang R, Yuan S, et al. Quality of life after surgical resection compared with radiofrequency ablation for small hepatocellular carcinomas. The British Journal of Surgery. 2014;**101**:1006-1015

[56] Salem R, Gilbertsen M, Butt Z, Memon K, Vouche M, Hickey R, et al. Increased quality of life among hepatocellular carcinoma patients treated with radioembolization, compared with chemoembolization. Clinical Gastroenterology Hepatology. 2013;**11**:1358-1365

Chapter 7

Long-Term Toxicities among Wilms Tumor Survivors

Samir Patel, Andrea Lo, Luke E. Pater, Mary Frances McAleer, Arnold Paulino and John A. Kalapurakal

Abstract

Successive trials conducted by the National Wilms Tumor Study have resulted in very high cure rates for children with Wilms tumor (WT). These trials have also significantly reduced the indications for doxorubicin and higher doses of RT in WT. Late toxicities after multimodality treatment especially RT, continues to be a major problem among WT survivors. Higher doses of RT is the most important factor responsible for the many late effects including congestive heart failure, secondary malignant neoplasms, hypogonadism, infertility and pregnancy complications, pulmonary disease, musculoskeletal effects, renal failure and diabetes mellitus. The potential for novel RT techniques like IMRT and proton therapy to reduce the incidence of these toxicities is discussed. The surveillance recommendations for WT survivors are mainly derived from the COG long-term follow-up guidelines. The future directions in late effects research include novel research to improve current knowledge of association between RT doses to target organs and late effects, discovery of novel biomarkers, and identification of predictive genetic biomarkers. Despite all these advances, there are significant challenges facing the global health care community that need to be overcome before the benefits of these innovations in late effects research can be translated to individual cancer survivors.

Keywords: Wilms tumor, radiation therapy, survivors, late toxicities, surveillance, prevention

1. Introduction

Successive trials conducted by the National Wilms Tumor Study (NWTS) have led to major improvements in the overall survival of children afflicted with Wilms tumor (WT). These trials have also been successful in reducing the indications for and dosages of radiation therapy (RT) and doxorubicin in the majority of children with WT. However, late toxicity of treatment continues to be a concern with radiation therapy (RT) as a major contributor [1]. Organs in the abdomen such as the liver, pancreas, spleen and bowel may be included in the flank RT field. For whole abdominal RT (WART), in addition to these organs, the remaining kidney, uterus and the ovaries are included in the RT field, and the testicles and breast tissue receiving scatter radiation. The heart, lungs, thyroid gland and breast tissue are at risk for late effects when whole lung irradiation (WLI) is utilized.

The bone, muscles and soft tissues are also at risk for growth disturbances when the abdomen and/or chest are irradiated. Finally, there is a potential risk of secondary malignant neoplasms in all of these organs exposed to any dose of RT.

Long-term follow up of the NWTS cohort showed that the standardized mortality ratio (SMR) was 24.3 for the first 5 years, 12.6 for the next 5 years, and remained greater than 3.0 thereafter. Secondary malignant neoplasms and congestive heart failure (CHF) were the commonest causes of long-term mortality [2]. Likewise, in the Childhood Cancer Survival Study (CCSS), the overall survival rate at 25 years after diagnosis of WT was 93.9%. The overall SMR was 4.9, and SMR for survivors who received abdominal and chest RT without doxorubicin was 6.1, and with doxorubicin the SMR was 12.3. Also, the cumulative incidence of chronic health conditions at 25 years after diagnosis was 65.4% and that of severe conditions (grades 3 to 5) was 24.2%. WT survivors had twice the rate of grades 1 to 4 chronic health conditions (Hazard Ratio [HR] 2.0) and 4.7 times higher rates of severe chronic health conditions (grades 3 or 4) (HR 4.7) than the sibling comparison group [3].

Children with WT are typically young, as the median age at initial presentation is between 3 to 4 years; hence, any reduction in RT dose and volume may have an impact on lowering treatment complications. RT dose reduction from 40 to 10 Gy in Stage III FH and the omission of WLI in Stage IV FH WT patients with isolated pulmonary metastases, favorable biology and complete response to chemotherapy are some of the strategies that have been used in the NWTS and Children's Oncology Group (COG) to minimize RT late effects [4, 5]. The use of more modern techniques of RT delivery such as intensity modulated radiation therapy (IMRT) and proton therapy can likewise potentially reduce RT complications. This chapter will examine the acute and late RT toxicities observed in Wilms tumor patients as well as some of the strategies that have been employed to minimize long-term complications.

2. Cardiac toxicity

Cardiotoxicity, specifically congestive heart failure (CHF) is a leading cause of morbidity and mortality in long-term survivors of Wilms tumor [2, 3]. Anthracyclines have preferential myocytic toxicity that results in a reduction of myocardial mass, myofibril dysfunction, decrease in contractility, and cardiomyopathy [6]. The most important risk factor is cumulative anthracycline dose, although all dose levels have been associated with myocyte injury [7]. Asymptomatic echocardiographic abnormalities such as increased end-systolic wall stress or decreased contractility can be found in survivors [8, 9]. Further, cardiac damage from therapy is progressive with an increasing lifelong risk of developing cardiac dysfunction that may necessitate cardiac transplant in some survivors [10, 11]. The severity of late cardiac effects will depend on factors including the age and sex of the child at time of treatment, cumulative anthracycline dose, cardiac radiation exposure, and presence of independent risk factors for cardiovascular disease not related to therapy.

Cardiac irradiation may result in scarring and stiffening of heart tissues resulting in arrhythmias, cardiomyopathy, valvular stenosis or insufficiency, coronary artery disease, and pericarditis or pericardial fibrosis [12]. Risk factors for cardiac morbidity include patient age at time of RT, RT dose and fractionation, irradiated cardiac volume, exposure to chemotherapeutic agents, and presence of cardiovascular risk factors.

The 20-year cumulative frequency of CHF among patients on NWTS-1 to NWTS-4 studies was 4.4% in patients initially treated with doxorubicin and 17.4%

in patients treated with doxorubicin for first or subsequent relapse [13]. The relative risk (RR) of CHF was increased with female sex (relative risk RR 4.5) and cumulative doxorubicin dose (RR 3.2/100 mg/m2), and left abdominal RT (RR 1.8/10 Gy). In an analysis of patients enrolled on the NWTS-3 and NWTS-4 studies, the 20-year risk of CHF after primary treatment with doxorubicin was 1.2% [14]. In a report from the CCSS, after 25 years of follow up, the HRs were 23.6 for CHF, 50.7 for renal failure, and 8.2 for hypertension (HTN), compared to the sibling group. Exposure to doxorubicin, in the absence of cardiac RT, did not show a clear association with an increased risk of CHF (≤ 250 mg/m2, HR 4.8). Cardiac RT was associated with an elevated risk of developing CHF. In the absence of doxorubicin, cardiac RT was associated with a HR of 6.6 for CHF. The HR for CHF was increased among those who received both cardiac RT and doxorubicin (≤ 250 mg/m2, HR 13.0, > 250 mg/m2, HR 18.3) [3].

The first study to corelate mean cardiac dose with late cardiac morbidity was a study of 4122 five-year French and British childhood survivors (mean follow-up, 27 years). The risk of cardiac death was higher in patients who received a mean cardiac RT dose of >5 Gy (5–14.9 Gy RR 12.5; >15 Gy RR, 25.1) and cumulative anthracycline dose of >360 mg/m2 (RR 4.4). There was a linear relationship between the mean cardiac RT dose and the risk of cardiac death (adjusted RR at 1 Gy, 60%) [15]. In another report of 229 childhood cancer survivors at the Institute Gustave Roussy 15 years or more after doxorubicin therapy, patients who received a mean cardiac RT dose between 5 and 20 Gy had a RR of CHF of 2.52 and those who received ≥20 Gy had a RR 5.65. The 25-year risk of cardiac failure was estimated at 34% in the 34 patients who received ≥250 mg/m2 of doxorubicin and mean cardiac RT dose of ≥5 Gy [16]. A report from the CCSS showed a dose-response relationship between mean cardiac RT dose and any cardiac disease, coronary artery disease and heart failure at mean doses ≥10 Gy. Exposure of low- to moderate-dose RT (5 to 19 Gy) to a large volume of the heart (≥ 50%) had a 1.6-fold increased risk of cardiac disease and exposure of any volume of the heart to RT doses of ≥20 Gy conferred an increased risk of cardiac disease [17].

3. Mitigation strategies and surveillance guidelines

The use of two parallel-opposed anterior-posterior (AP) and posterior-anterior (PA) fields has been the conventional approach for RT of WT for many decades. Modern RT techniques such as cardiac sparing whole lung intensity-modulated radiation therapy (IMRT) techniques haves been shown statistically significant reduction of cardiac and myocardial RT doses compared to standard AP-PA WLI techniques in a prospective clinical trial [12]. Another report showed that the mean cardiac dose was significantly higher when the lung and abdomen RT fields were treated sequentially compared to when they were treated concurrently [18]. All current and future COG protocols will permit the use of cardiac sparing whole lung IMRT with central quality assurance review, concurrent treatment of lung and abdomen RT fields and IMRT/proton therapy for the treatment of flank and whole abdomen.

The COG LTFU guidelines, version 5.0, provide extensive recommendations for the appropriate surveillance of childhood cancer survivors for common RT-induced toxicities observed in WT survivors (http://survivorshipguidelines.org). A summary of these guidelines is provided in **Table 1**.

	Anthracycline Dose	Radiation Dose	Recommendation
Medical history	All survivors		Evaluate for: shortness of breath, dyspnea on exertion, orthopnea, palpitations, chest pain
	Survivors aged <25 years		Abdominal symptoms (nausea, vomiting)
Physical Examination and Counseling	All survivors		Yearly blood pressure and cardiac examination Maintain appropriate weight, blood pressure and heart-healthy diet. Regular exercise should be encouraged for patients who have normal LV systolic function. High-risk survivors should consult with a cardiologist to define limits and precautions for physical activity For female patients who are pregnant or planning to become pregnant, additional cardiology evaluation is indicated in patients who received: ≥250 mg/m2 anthracyclines— ≥ 35 Gy chest radiation, or— Anthracycline (any dose) combined with chest radiation (≥15 Gy)
Echocardiogram	None	< 15 Gy	Not required
	None	≥ 15 Gy and < 35 Gy	Every 5 years
	None	≥ 35 Gy	Every 2 years
	< 250 mg/m2	< 15 Gy	Every 5 years
	< 250 mg/m2	≥ 15 Gy	Every 2 years
	≥ 250 mg/m2		Every 2 years
Electrocardiogram	All survivors		Baseline and as needed thereafter

Table 1.
The Children's oncology group long-term follow-up guidelines recommendations (summary) for surveillance of childhood cancer survivors exposed to anthracycline therapy (http://survivorshipguidelines.org).

4. Secondary malignant neoplasms

With the increase in survivorship in children with WT, there has been an accompanying increase in secondary malignant neoplasms (SMN). Among long-term WT survivors in the CCSS cohort, the cumulative incidence of SMN was 3.0% at 25 years. The most common SMNs were soft tissue sarcomas which occurred in six survivors. Five WT survivors had confirmed breast cancer. RT exposure of the breast in these patients ranged from 13 to 17.5 Gy. There were four bone tumors: two osteogenic sarcomas; one Ewing sarcoma; and one other bone tumor. The other SMNs were four adenocarcinomas, three melanoma, three thyroid cancers, two lymphoid leukemias, one medulloblastoma, and seven other cancers including one secondary renal cell carcinoma. SMNs were the most common cause of death in long-term WT survivors [3]. A SEER database review noted an incidence of SMN in patients treated for WT at 0.6% at 10 years, increasing to 1.6% at 20 years and 3.8% at 30 years [19]. A combined cohort study of patients from the NWTS, CCSS British and Nordic national registries provided data on 13,351 subjects diagnosed under the age of 15 in 1960 or later followed for a median of 11.6 years. After 169,641 person-years (PY) of observation through 2005, 174 solid tumors (exclusive of basal cell carcinomas) and 28 leukemias were ascertained in 195 subjects. Age-specific incidence of secondary solid tumors increased from approximately 1 case per 1000 PY at age 15 to 5 cases per 1000 PY at age 40. The cumulative incidence of solid tumors at age 40 was 6.7%. Leukemia risk, by contrast, was highest during the first 5 years following WT diagnosis. The Standardized incidence ratios (SIRs) for solid tumors and leukemias were 5.1 and 5.0, respectively. Among solid tumors, the most common were cancers of the digestive organs, most commonly hepatocellular carcinoma with 8 cases. There were 23 cases of breast cancer, 15 thyroid cancers and 11 osteosarcomas. There was a demonstrated difference in the observed incidence over time. At 10 years from diagnosis, the incidence was 1 SMN per 1000 survivors per year which increased to 5–6 solid tumors per 1000 survivors per year by 35 years after diagnosis. Also noted was a 49% increase in standardized incidence ratio (SIR) for SMN for patients diagnosed and treated after the age of 5 years. The occurrence of a solid SMN dramatically affected survival prospects [20]. The Mayo Clinic reported on 8295 patients treated from 1970 to 2020 for pediatric cancers. Eleven patients were identified to have developed subsequent renal neoplasms. Six of these eleven were patients previously treated for WT with clear cell sarcoma being the most common secondary renal cancer [21].

The use of RT and doxorubicin has been clearly associated with higher risk of SMNs. In the British Childhood Cancer Survivor Study, the majority of solid tumors (35 of 39, 89.7%) of the thorax, abdomen or pelvis developed within irradiated fields [22]. In the NWTS series, RT increased the risk of a SMN (SIR, 1.43/10 Gy) and doxorubicin potentiated the RT effect. Among 234 patients who received doxorubicin and > 35 Gy of abdominal RT, the SIR was 36. The changes in RT doses in NWTS protocols from 40 Gy in the 1960s to 10 Gy in the 1990s was also associated with a decrease in time-specific incidence rates of SMNs [23].

Due to the utilization of WLI in the management of WT with lung metastases, the incidence of breast cancer in WT survivors is significantly increased compared to the general population. A report from the NWTS reported the incidence and risk factors for breast cancer among 2492 female patients treated from 1969 to 1995. There were 29 cases of invasive breast cancer and 6 cases of ductal carcinoma in-situ, representing a SIR of 9.1 for invasive disease and cumulative risk at age 40 (CR40) of 4.5%. Among women who had chest RT, the SIR was 27.6 and CR40 was 14.8%. The majority of patients received 12Gy. WART was associated with a SIR of 7.2 and flank only RT had a SIR of 5.8. The CR40 was 3.1% for female patients who received abdominal RT. Patients not undergoing RT had a SIR of 2.2., The SIR for DCIS in patients undergoing chest or abdominal RT was 9.2, comparable to that for invasive disease [24]. Subsequent analysis of this data set included an assessment of male breast cancer and no excess risk was identified [25]. Among 20,276 CCSS survivors of which 6498 women were eligible for analysis, 95 women had 111 confirmed cases of breast cancer. The majority (65 patients) were treated for Hodgkin lymphoma. Only 3 patients were treated for WT with 2 of the 3 cases receiving chest RT [26].

5. Mitigation strategies and surveillance guidelines

A number of strategies including avoidance of RT and the use of lower doses of RT in modern COG and SIOP protocols may reduce the risk of SMNs. SIOP 93-01 allowed for omission of WLI in patients achieving radiographic CR of lung metastases following 6 weeks of chemotherapy or undergoing resection of all residual lung disease. Only 14%

	Factors that may increase risk	Recommendation
Breast Cancer	Patient factors: Family history of breast cancer. Personal history of BRCA1, BRCA2, ATM or p53 mutation or in absence of personal genetic testing, known BRCA mutation in first degree relative Treatment factors: Higher RT dose, especially ≥10 Gy, longer time since radiation (>5 years).	Yearly, beginning at puberty until age 25, then every 6 months. Teach breast self-exam and counsel to perform monthly beginning at puberty. Mammogram yearly, beginning 8 years after radiation or at age 25, whichever occurs last. Breast MRI yearly, as an adjunct to mammography beginning 8 years after radiation or at age 25, whichever occurs last
Colorectal Cancer screening (Stool multitarget DNA test)		Beginning 5 years after radiation or at age 30 years (whichever occurs last). Every 3 years. Positive result should be followed up with timely colonoscopy.
Thyroid cancer	Patient factors: Younger age at treatment Treatment factors: >5 years after RT, highest risk is between 10 and 30 Gy, thyroid gland directly in RT field, Total Body Irradiation, alkylating agents	Thyroid exam Yearly Ultrasound for evaluation of palpable nodule(s). FNA as clinically indicated. Endocrine and/or surgical consultation for further management.

Table 2.
The Children's oncology group long-term follow-up guidelines (summary) recommendations for surveillance of childhood cancer survivors for secondary malignancy.

of patients required lung RT as upfront therapy with this approach with good survival outcomes [27]. Similarly in COG AREN0533 trial, good survival rates were observed after omission of WLI in children whose tumors were without LOH at 1p and 16q and had complete response of lung nodules following chemotherapy at 6 weeks [28].

The International Guideline Harmonization Group updated their breast cancer surveillance recommendations in 2020. They noted that current data showed correlation between more moderate doses of RT (10–19Gy) and the risk of breast cancer. Additionally, there was a relationship between the use of anthracyclines and risk of breast cancer. Taking into account the risks of increased surveillance and relative benefit, the primary changes to previous recommendations were for surveillance for female patients with exposures of 10Gy or more to the chest, upper abdominal RT exposing the breast tissue at a young age and the use of anthracyclines [29].

The COG LTFU guidelines, version 5.0, provide extensive recommendations for the appropriate surveillance of childhood cancer survivors for common RT-induced toxicities observed in WT survivors (http://survivorshipguidelines.org). A summary of these guidelines is provided in **Table 2**.

6. Hypogonadism, infertility and pregnancy complications

WT is predominantly diagnosed in prepubertal children, with the incidence peaking at 12 months in males and 12–36 months in females, and is among the few malignancies that occurs more frequently in females than males [30]. With current therapeutic regimens that include the of large chest and flank/ WART fields, it is important to consider the impact of these treatments on gonadal function and reproduction in WT survivors. The potential RT exposure of the gonads can range from internal scattered doses only (e.g., flank RT) to full RT dose (e.g., whole abdomen [WART] in females).

6.1 Impact of RT on fertility in males with WT

Early reports of small numbers of male survivors of WT identified primary gonadal failure following 15–30 Gy flank or WART at 0.5–4 years of age [31] as well as reduced gonadal volume and sperm production after 2.7–9.8 Gy testicular dose after WART [32]. Of note, these findings were attributed to RT as chemotherapy did not show any such effects. An analysis of over 6000 male childhood cancer survivors, of which 429 had WT, revealed RT >7.5 Gy to the testes significantly reduced the ability to father children compared to survivors with no radiation exposure [33].

6.2 Impact of RT on fertility and gestation in females with WT

As noted for male patients, studies have also shown female patients to have primary gonadal failure following 15–30 Gy flank or WART at 0.5–4 years of age [31]. Another study showed atrophied ipsilateral ovary in half of those treated with 4–41 Gy to the flank and atrophied bilateral ovaries in all patients treated with 21–30 Gy WART prior to puberty [34]. In addition to potential impact on gonadal function, late effects of RT to the abdominopelvic region in young children may impair normal growth and development of the irradiated pelvic bones, vasculature and organs including the uterus that are essential for successful gestation. Early studies of pregnancy outcomes in irradiated female WT survivors have shown increased incidence of perinatal death, low birthweight, and birth defects compared with offspring of unirradiated female survivors, sibling controls or wives of male WT survivors, regardless of chemotherapy exposure [35, 36]. In an analysis of 309 female WT survivors treated on NWTS 1–4, flank RT >25 Gy was associated with significantly increased risk of preterm labor, fetal malposition and lower mean gestational age with odds ratio of 2.36, 6.26 and 4.07, respectively compared to unirradiated female survivors [37]. This effect was not observed for female survivors receiving chemotherapy only or for gestations fathered by male survivors. In a subset of 126 of these female WT survivors who received more than flank RT, only seven were able to conceive at least once. Five of these women received upper abdominal RT, with nine of 10 gestations resulting in live births; the remaining two women received WART, with the one receiving 10.5 Gy able to have a single viable birth and the other receiving 21 Gy having three non-viable pregnancies [38].

7. Mitigation strategies and surveillance guidelines

Given the young age of most WT patients, it is imperative to counsel caregivers of the late fertility risks of therapy and to involve endocrinology specialists early in the care of these patients [39]. With the continued advances in novel biomarker discovery and revised tumor-risk based stratifications, RT technology, including improvements in image-guidance and increased availability of proton beam therapy, it may be possible to further reduce radiation exposure to organs-at-risk involved in fertility and gestation and thereby reduce the undesired late effects of RT on fertility in WT survivors.

	Factors that may increase risk	Recommendation
Ovarian dysfunction	The ovaries are included in flank/hemiabdomen RT fields only if the fields extended below iliac crest. Patient factors: Older age at RT Treatment factors: RT dose ≥5 Gy if pubertal (especially dose ≥10 Gy), RT dose ≥10 Gy if prepubertal (especially dose ≥15 Gy), combination with alkylating agent chemotherapy, longer time since treatment, combination with cyclophosphamide conditioning for high dose chemotherapy regimens.	Yearly evaluation for: Onset and tempo of puberty Menstrual history Sexual function (vaginal dryness, libido) Menopausal symptoms Medication use Sexual function (vaginal dryness, libido) Menopausal symptoms Medication use Tanner staging until sexually mature Yearly Monitor growth until mature FSH and estradiol and/or endocrine/gynecology referral for patients with no signs of puberty at age 13, failure of pubertal progression, abnormal menstrual patterns or menopausal symptoms. Bone density evaluation in patients with ovarian hormone deficiencies.
Reduced ovarian follicular pool Infertility	The ovaries are included in the left and right flank RT fields only if they extended below iliac crest. Patient factors: Older age at RT Treatment factors: RT dose ≥5 Gy if pubertal (especially dose ≥10 Gy), RT dose ≥10 Gy if prepubertal (especially dose ≥15 Gy), combination with alkylating agent chemotherapy, longer time since treatment, combination with cyclophosphamide conditioning for high dose chemotherapy regimens.	Yearly evaluation for: Menstrual and pregnancy history Hormonal Therapy Tanner staging until sexually mature FSH and estradiol for patients with menstrual cycle dysfunction suggestive of premature ovarian insufficiency or those who desire information about potential for future fertility. AMH (anti-Mullerian hormone) to assess for diminished ovarian reserve. Reproductive endocrinology referral for assisted reproductive and interventions to preserve future fertility.
Uterine vascular insufficiency resulting in adverse pregnancy outcomes like spontaneous abortion, neonatal death, low-birth weight infant, fetal malposition and premature labor	The uterus is included in the left and right flank RT fields only if they extended below iliac crest. Patient factors: Wilms tumor and associated Müllerian anomalies, prepubertal at time of treatment Treatment factors: Total body Irradiation, higher RT dose to pelvis, or RT dose ≥30 Gy	Yearly evaluation for: Pregnancy and Childbirth history High-level ultrasound evaluation of genitourinary tract after pubertal development as clinically indicated in patients contemplating pregnancy. High-risk obstetrical care during pregnancy
Pulmonary Toxicity	Patient factors: Younger age at RT. Pre-morbid/Co-morbid medical conditions: Atopic history—Health behaviors: Smoking, inhaled illicit drug use Treatment factors: RT dose >10 Gy, especially RT dose ≥15 Gy, Total body Irradiation ≥6 Gy in single fraction, TBI ≥12 Gy fractionated, RT combined with bleomycin, busulfan, carmustine (BCNU), or lomustine (CCNU), radiomimetic chemotherapy (e.g., doxorubicin, dactinomycin)	Clinical Pulmonary exam Yearly PFTs (including DLCO and spirometry) Baseline at entry into long-term follow-up, repeat as clinically indicated. Repeat PFTs prior to general anesthesia. Influenza and Pneumococcal vaccinations.

DOI: http://dx.doi.org/10.5772/intechopen.110130

	Factors that may increase risk	Recommendation
Musculoskeletal growth problems: Hypoplasia, fibrosis, Kyphosis, Scoliosis	Patient factors: Younger age at treatment, especially prepubertal at treatment Treatment factors: Higher RT dose, especially dose ≥20 Gy, larger RT field, higher radiation dose per fraction, orthovoltage radiation	Yearly Height Weight Sitting height for patients who had trunk radiation Orthopedic consultation for any deficit noted in growing child. Plastic surgery consult for reconstruction.
Renal dysfunction	Patient factors: congenital syndromes (WAGR, DDS, hypospadias, cryptorchidism), Diabetes mellitus, hypertension, congenital absence of kidney Treatment factors: Bilateral Wilms tumor, nephrectomy, radiomimetic chemotherapy (e.g., doxorubicin, dactinomycin), combination with other nephrotoxic agents (e.g., cisplatin, carboplatin, ifosfamide, aminoglycosides, amphotericin, immunosuppressants), RT dose ≥10 Gy, especially RT dose ≥15 Gy, TBI ≥6 Gy in single fraction, TBI ≥12 Gy fractionated, TBI combined with radiation to the kidney	Blood pressure Yearly BUN Creatinine Na, K, Cl, CO2, Ca, Mg, PO4 Baseline at entry into long-term follow-up, repeat as clinically indicated.
Diabetes Mellitus Impaired glucose metabolism may occur as part of a metabolic syndrome that includes central obesity with at least 2 or more of the following: hypertension, atherogenic dyslipidemia, and abnormal glucose metabolism.	Patient factors: Family history of diabetes mellitus, Obesity Treatment factors: Abdomen RT, TBI Prolonged corticosteroid therapy	Fasting blood glucose OR HbA1c Every 2 years Diet and Physical Activity Cardiovascular Risk Factors Endocrine consultation Evaluate for other co-morbid conditions, including dyslipidemia, hypertension, and overweight/obesity. Refer to dietician for blood sugar management.

Table 3.
The Children's oncology group long-term follow-up guidelines recommendations for surveillance of childhood cancer survivors for common RT-induced toxicities observed in WT survivors.

The International Late Effects of Childhood Cancer Guideline Harmonization Group have recently published evidence-based consensus recommendations for fertility preservation, including testicular and ovarian cryopreservation, in young cancer patients [40]. Currently, fertility preservation for WT patients is largely experimental, expensive and not widely available. Most patients are prepubertal, and there are no established criteria and standard guidelines for fertility preservation in males and ovarian cryopreservation in prepubertal females. Clinicians should proactively initiate conversations around standard and experimental options for fertility preservation in high risk WT children. Other options that exist for WT survivors of both genders include adoption, surrogacy, and the use of donor sperm/eggs or embryos.

The COG LTFU guidelines, version 5.0, provide extensive recommendations for the appropriate surveillance of childhood cancer survivors for common RT-induced toxicities observed in WT survivors (http://survivorshipguidelines.org). A summary of these guidelines is provided in **Table 3**.

8. Pulmonary disease

Pulmonary disease is an uncommon but important late effect observed in survivors of WT. In a report from the NWTS on 6449 survivors WT survivors from NWTS 1–4 after a median follow up of 17.9 years, 64 fully evaluable and 16 partially evaluable cases of pulmonary disease were identified. The 15-year cumulative incidence of pulmonary disease was 4.0% among fully evaluable and 4.8%among fully and partially evaluable patients who received WLI for pulmonary metastases at initial diagnosis. In contrast, 15-year cumulative incidence of pulmonary disease was much lower (<0.5%) among those who did not receive WLI. Survivors who had lung RT for relapse treatment had higher rates of pulmonary disease than those who had lung RT at initial treatment (hazard ratio [HR] 1.7). Survivors who received abdominal RT only had higher rates than those who received no RT at all (HR 3.5) [41]. Foster et al. reported on 280 WT survivors compared to 625 age and sex-matched controls for childhood cancer from St. Jude Children's Hospital [42]. At a median follow up of 26 years, compared to controls, survivors had an excess grade 2 to 4 obstructive (11.7 vs. 2.9%, $P < 0.01$), restrictive (9.6 vs. 0.2%, $P < 0.01$), and diffusion (10.4 vs. 0.3%, $P < 0.01$) pulmonary impairments. Adjusting for smoking status, pulmonary diffusion defects were associated with doxorubicin (RR 3.9) and restrictive deficits with chest radiation (RR 12.3).

9. Mitigation strategies and surveillance guidelines

The avoidance of lung RT in children with good response to chemotherapy and lack of adverse biomarkers can significantly reduce the risks for pulmonary toxicity. Modern protocols with IMRT in COG use lower doses of RT (12Gy) with lung heterogeneity compared to SIOP protocols.

The COG LTFU guidelines, version 5.0, provide extensive recommendations for the appropriate surveillance of childhood cancer survivors for common RT-induced toxicities observed in WT survivors (http://survivorshipguidelines.org). A summary of these guidelines is provided in **Table 3**.

10. Musculoskeletal effects

Musculoskeletal toxicity may occur from RT in young children, the severity of which depends on the patient's age at treatment, RT dose, fractionation and RT fields. Growth of normal tissues can be impaired, resulting in reduced spinal growth and sitting height after RT for WT [43]. Scoliosis and kyphosis are other possible complications WT therapy, which may be a result of reactive myocontracture and shortened soft tissues from RT [44, 45], or nerve injury related to surgery [46]. At a median follow-up of 12–13 years, WT survivors have reported scoliosis in 54–67% and kyphosis in 14%, with 10–20% experiencing symptoms or requiring intervention [46, 47]. A higher scoliosis rate of 88% was observed by Mäkipernaa et al., potentially related to a longer median follow-up of 19 years and more complete radiologic follow-up; nevertheless, the vast majority of patients were still mild and asymptomatic, with 3 of 21 having a scoliosis curvature greater than 10° and only 1 being symptomatic. It is noteworthy that the available data on musculoskeletal complications involved WT patients treated to higher RT doses (median doses >30Gy) than are typically used in the current era [46–48]. Thus, it is likely that the incidence and severity of scoliosis after modern WT therapy are lower than previously published. Slipped femoral capital epiphyses can occur after RT for WT that includes the hip joint. The incidence is higher in children <4 years of age and after RT doses >25 Gy to the hip [49].

11. Mitigation strategies and surveillance guidelines

A number of strategies including avoidance of RT, use of lower doses of RT (10–20Gy) in modern COG and SIOP protocols, inclusion of the entire vertebral body during RT and blocking the hip joint completely can reduce musculoskeletal toxicity among WT survivors.

The COG LTFU guidelines, version 5.0, provide extensive recommendations for the appropriate surveillance of childhood cancer survivors for common RT-induced toxicities observed in WT survivors (http://survivorshipguidelines.org). A summary of these guidelines is provided in **Table 3**.

12. Renal failure

Renal function is an important consideration in survivors of WT, particularly in those who develop progression of bilateral WT or receive RT to the opposite kidney in unilateral disease. Non-syndromic children with unilateral WT treated with radical nephrectomy without nephrotoxic chemotherapy or RT are at low risk for significant long-term renal dysfunction [50]. Although a significant number of survivors have subclinical glomerular and tubular damage [51, 52], the risk of end-stage renal disease (ESRD) is very low in most patients with unilateral WT. A study on 5910 patients enrolled in NWTS showed that the 20-year cumulative incidence of end-stage renal disease (ESRD) after unilateral WT was 74% in children with Denys Drash syndrome, 36% in children with WAGR syndrome, 7% in male patients with hypospadias or cryptorchidism and 0.6% in non-syndromic WT patients. Twenty-year cumulative incidence of ESRD after bilateral Wilms tumor was 50% in children with Denys Drash syndrome, 90% in children with WAGR syndrome, 25% in male patients with hypospadias and cryptorchidism and 12% in other non-syndromic patients [53]. A subsequent NWTS study assessed risk factors for ESRD in those without known WT1-related syndromes; it was found that patients with characteristics associated with a WT1 etiology (stromal predominant histology, intralobar nephrogenic rests and WT diagnosis at <24 months) had a higher risk of ESRD due to chronic renal failure [54]. In other reports from the CCSS and Denmark, renal tumor survivors after 18–20 years after treatment with nephrectomy and abdominal RT, had good renal function based on estimated glomerular filtration rates, although eGFR was significantly lower than in the normal population. WT survivors also had higher rates of albuminuria and hypertension [55, 56].

13. Mitigation strategies and surveillance guidelines

A number of strategies including avoidance of RT, use of lower doses of RT and modern RT technologies including IMRT and proton therapy may reduce the risks of renal toxicity in WT survivors.

The COG LTFU guidelines, version 5.0, provide extensive recommendations for the appropriate surveillance of childhood cancer survivors for common RT-induced toxicities observed in WT survivors (http://survivorshipguidelines.org). A summary of these guidelines is provided in **Table 3**.

14. Diabetes mellitus

The increased risk of diabetes mellitus (DM) from abdominal RT has been increasingly recognized over the past two decades, the pathophysiology of which is not completely clear, but likely related to the damage of insulin-producing ß cells concentrated in the tail of the pancreas [57]. In a study of Scandinavian childhood cancer survivors, the relative risks for DM were significantly increased in patients with WT, with an observed-to-expected first hospitalizations for DM of 2.9 [58]. A report from the Childhood Cancer Survivor Study demonstrated that WT survivors were more likely to be diabetic than siblings (RR 3.77), and this association remained significant when adjusted for body mass index. Among cancer survivors treated with abdominal RT, greater attained age, higher body mass index and increasing pancreatic tail dose were associated with increased DM risk [59]. In addition, a statistically significant interaction was noted between younger age at cancer diagnosis and mean pancreatic tail dose, with greater differences in DM risk noted among those diagnosed at the youngest ages. Among survivors diagnosed at age 5 years, relative risk of DM was 2.98 after a mean pancreatic dose of 10–19.9 Gy, 3.62, after 20–29.9 Gy, and 4.66 after 30+ Gy, with reference group being 0.1–9.9 Gy [59].

15. Mitigation strategies and surveillance guidelines

A number of strategies including avoidance of RT, use of lower doses of RT and modern RT technologies including IMRT and proton therapy may reduce the risks of diabetes mellitus among WT survivors.

The COG LTFU guidelines, version 5.0, provide extensive recommendations for the appropriate surveillance of childhood cancer survivors for common RT-induced toxicities observed in WT survivors (http://survivorshipguidelines.org). A summary of these guidelines is provided in **Table 3**.

16. Conclusions and future directions

The cure rates of WT patients following multimodality therapy including RT are excellent. However, RT is an important cause of late toxicity. Novel RT techniques such as IMRT for abdominal and lung RT and proton therapy are currently being studied in SIOP and COG in prospective clinical trials and may reduce the incidence of late toxicity. Currently WT biomarkers are only utilized for defining high-risk tumors to be treated with chemotherapy. Their utilization for potentially refining indications for RT in certain risk groups remains to be studied. Detailed studies of late toxicities specifically by analyzing the effects of RT doses to target organs is critical to improve our understanding of the relationship between RT and a variety of toxicities such as infertility, hypogonadism, congestive heart failure and secondary malignancies [60]. International collaborations like the Pediatric Normal Tissue Effects in the Clinic (PENTEC), are systematically analyzing the association between RT doses and volumes and organ toxicities by reviewing published reports of late toxicities following RT in children. However, a large number of reports lack detailed RT doses and organ dose-volume correlations for these reported toxicities. Another approach, as used by the CCSS, is to perform retrospective dosimetry using patient age and sex-matched phantoms to recreate multiorgan dosimetry from past treatments for correlation with late toxicities [61]. A similar approach using patient-matched 3D University of Florida/National Cancer Institute (UF/NCI) phantoms is currently being completed by the NWTS Late Effects Study [60]. A better understanding of the RT dose thresholds for these toxicities will help promote the adoption of interventions for their prevention and mitigation. The revision of previous RT dose thresholds (>20 Gy) for breast cancer surveillance to 12 Gy following reports by the NWTS is an important example of the critical value of such studies [62].

There are many preclinical and clinical reports that describe novel biomarkers that could detect RT injury in various organs more accurately and earlier in the time course after treatment. These biomarkers could greatly improve our understanding of risks of RT and refine surveillance guidelines for high-risk survivors to mitigate late toxicity [63, 64]. Another area of importance that deserves further study is the assessment of risk for late toxicities based on individualized genetic susceptibility to cancer treatment. Currently, while there are no established genetic biomarkers for RT induced toxicities, there are few reports of large-scale genome wide association studies (GWAS) that have identified several single nucleotide polymorphisms (SNPs), linked to breast cancer after RT exposure, cardiovascular toxicity and ovarian failure after cancer therapy [65–67]. The identification of predictive genetic biomarkers that may interact with RT or chemotherapy and increase the likelihood of these toxicities may permit individualized treatment and surveillance guidelines to minimize these risks and maximize long-term quality of life. Currently, the NIH is providing funding opportunities to advance understanding of mechanistic interactions and biologic consequences of RT prioritizing a comprehensive study of patient (genomic and epigenomics), tumor and treatment (chemotherapy, RT, dosimetry) factors, together with longitudinal multiomics (pre and post-therapy) to improve our understanding of the effects of RT on normal tissues (RFA-CA-21-040). Such novel studies could lead to the discovery of new biomarkers and novel therapeutics that could mitigate RT induced complications and improve tumor control rates in children with cancer.

Despite all these advances, there are significant challenges facing health care providers in their efforts to improve the long-term health and quality of life of childhood cancer survivors. The Academy of Medicine (AOM) recommends that cancer survivors be provided survivorship care plans (SCPs) that include treatment summaries and follow-up plans [68]. The '*Passport for Care®*' (PFC) program is a free interactive internet resource for global use that addresses the need to provide childhood cancer survivors and primary care physicians with accurate and individualized health care information based on patients' age, sex, diagnosis, chemotherapy, RT, surgery, clinical history and other related data. The PFC program provides recommendations derived from the long-term COG follow-up guidelines [69]. However, SCPs have not been shown to improve patient reported outcomes due to notable barriers to routine implementation relating to health care providers and survivors such as lack of family and social support for survivors especially among minorities, lack of transition of care, lack of interest and knowledge among primary care providers, knowledge gap among survivors, lack of financial support and psychologic issues including addictions among survivors, among others [70–73]. All of these issues need to be addressed by the global medical community, and new health care models with improved collaboration, better coordination and more communication among survivors and their clinicians will be required to translate the benefits of many of these innovations in late effects research to individual childhood cancer survivors [68, 74].

Author details

Samir Patel[1], Andrea Lo[2], Luke E. Pater[3], Mary Frances McAleer[4], Arnold Paulino[4] and John A. Kalapurakal[5]*

1 Department of Radiation Oncology, Cross Cancer Institute, Edmonton, AB, Canada

2 Division of Radiation Oncology, University of British Columbia, Vancouver, BC, Canada

3 Department of Radiation Oncology, University of Cincinnati Medical Center, Cincinnati, OH, USA

4 Department of Radiation Oncology, University of Texas MD Anderson Cancer Center, Houston, TX, USA

5 Department of Radiation Oncology, Northwestern University Feinberg School of Medicine, Chicago, IL, USA

*Address all correspondence to: j-kalapurakal@northwestern.edu

References

[1] Dome JS, Mullen EA, Dix DB, Gratias EJ, Ehrlich PF, Daw NC, et al. Impact of the first generation of Children's oncology group clinical trials on clinical practice for Wilms tumor. Journal of the National Comprehensive Cancer Network. 2021;**19**(8):978-985

[2] Cotton CA, Peterson S, Norkool PA, Takashima J, Grigoriev Y, Green DM, et al. Early and late mortality after diagnosis of wilms tumor. Journal of Clinical Oncology. 2009;**27**(8):1304-1309

[3] Termuhlen AM, Tersak JM, Liu Q, Yasui Y, Stovall M, Weathers R, et al. Twenty-five year follow-up of childhood Wilms tumor: A report from the childhood cancer survivor study. Pediatric Blood & Cancer. 2011;**57**(7):1210-1216

[4] Thomas PR, Tefft M, Compaan PJ, Norkool P, Breslow NE, D'Angio GJ. Results of two radiation therapy randomizations in the third National Wilms' tumor study. Cancer. 1991;**68**(8):1703-1707

[5] Dix DB, Seibel NL, Chi YY, Khanna G, Gratias E, Anderson JR, et al. Treatment of stage IV favorable histology Wilms tumor with lung metastases: A report from the Children's oncology group AREN0533 study. Journal of Clinical Oncology. 2018;**36**(16):1564-1570

[6] Kaste SC, Dome JS, Babyn PS, Graf NM, Grundy P, Godzinski J, et al. Wilms tumour: Prognostic factors, staging, therapy and late effects. Pediatric Radiology. 2008;**38**(1):2-17

[7] Kremer LC, van der Pal HJ, Offringa M, van Dalen EC, Voute PA. Frequency and risk factors of subclinical cardiotoxicity after anthracycline therapy in children: A systematic review. Annals of Oncology. 2002;**13**(6):819-829

[8] Marx M, Langer T, Graf N, Hausdorf G, Stohr W, Ludwig R, et al. Multicentre analysis of anthracycline-induced cardiotoxicity in children following treatment according to the nephroblastoma studies SIOP No.9/GPOH and SIOP 93-01/GPOH. Medical and Pediatric Oncology. 2002;**39**(1):18-24

[9] Sorensen K, Levitt G, Sebag-Montefiore D, Bull C, Sullivan I. Cardiac function in Wilms' tumor survivors. Journal of Clinical Oncology. 1995;**13**(7):1546-1556

[10] Levitt G, Anazodo A, Burch M, Bunch K. Cardiac or cardiopulmonary transplantation in childhood cancer survivors: An increasing need? European Journal of Cancer. 2009;**45**(17):3027-3034

[11] Sorensen K, Levitt GA, Bull C, Dorup I, Sullivan ID. Late anthracycline cardiotoxicity after childhood cancer: A prospective longitudinal study. Cancer. 2003;**97**(8):1991-1998

[12] Kalapurakal JA, Gopalakrishnan M, Walterhouse DO, Rigsby CK, Rademaker A, Helenowski I, et al. Cardiac-sparing whole lung IMRT in patients with pediatric tumors and lung metastasis: Final report of a prospective multicenter clinical trial. International Journal of Radiation Oncology, Biology, Physics. 2019;**103**(1):28-37

[13] Green DM, Grigoriev YA, Nan B, Takashima JR, Norkool PA, D'Angio GJ, et al. Congestive heart failure after treatment for Wilms' tumor: A report from the National Wilms' tumor study group. Journal of Clinical Oncology. 2001;**19**(7):1926-1934

[14] Breslow NE, Ou SS, Beckwith JB, Haase GM, Kalapurakal JA, Ritchey ML, et al. Doxorubicin for favorable histology, stage II-III Wilms tumor: Results from the National Wilms Tumor Studies. Cancer. 2004;**101**(5):1072-1080

[15] Tukenova M, Guibout C, Oberlin O, Doyon F, Mousannif A, Haddy N, et al. Role of cancer treatment in long-term overall and cardiovascular mortality after childhood cancer. Journal of Clinical Oncology. 2010;**28**(8):1308-1315

[16] Pein F, Sakiroglu O, Dahan M, Lebidois J, Merlet P, Shamsaldin A, et al. Cardiac abnormalities 15 years and more after adriamycin therapy in 229 childhood survivors of a solid tumour at the Institut Gustave Roussy. British Journal of Cancer. 2004;**91**(1):37-44

[17] Bates JE, Howell RM, Liu Q, Yasui Y, Mulrooney DA, Dhakal S, et al. Therapy-related cardiac risk in childhood cancer survivors: An analysis of the childhood cancer survivor study. Journal of Clinical Oncology. 2019;**37**(13):1090-1101

[18] Farooqi A, Siddiqi A, Khan MK, Esiashvili N. Evaluation of radiation dose to cardiac and pulmonary tissue among patients with stage IV Wilms tumor and pulmonary metastases. Pediatric Blood & Cancer. 2014;**61**(8):1394-1397

[19] Lee JS, Padilla B, DuBois SG, Oates A, Boscardin J, Goldsby RE. Second malignant neoplasms among children, adolescents and young adults with Wilms tumor. Pediatric Blood & Cancer. 2015;**62**(7):1259-1264

[20] Breslow NE, Lange JM, Friedman DL, Green DM, Hawkins MM, Murphy MF, et al. Secondary malignant neoplasms after Wilms tumor: An international collaborative study. International Journal of Cancer. 2010;**127**(3):657-666

[21] Gupta S, Vanderbilt CM, Leibovich BC, Herrera-Hernandez L, Raghunathan A, Sukov WR, et al. Secondary renal neoplasia following chemotherapy or radiation in pediatric patients. Human Pathology. 2020;**103**:1-13

[22] Taylor AJ, Winter DL, Pritchard-Jones K, Stiller CA, Frobisher C, Lancashire ER, et al. Second primary neoplasms in survivors of Wilms' tumour—A population-based cohort study from the British childhood cancer survivor study. International Journal of Cancer. 2008;**122**(9):2085-2093

[23] Breslow NE, Takashima JR, Whitton JA, Moksness J, D'Angio GJ, Green DM. Second malignant neoplasms following treatment for Wilm's tumor: A report from the National Wilms' tumor study group. Journal of Clinical Oncology. 1995;**13**(8):1851-1859

[24] Lange J, Peterson SM, Takashima JR, Grigoriev Y, Ritchey ML, Shamberger RC, et al. Risk factors for end stage renal disease in non-wt1-syndromic wilms tumor. Journal of Urology. 2011;**186**(2):378-386

[25] Breslow NE, Peterson SM, Green DM. Reply to Wilms tumor and breast cancer. Cancer. 2015;**121**(12):2099-2100

[26] Kenney LB, Yasui Y, Inskip PD, Hammond S, Neglia JP, Mertens AC, et al. Breast cancer after childhood cancer: A report from the childhood cancer survivor study. Annals of Internal Medicine. 2004;**141**(8):590-597

[27] Verschuur A, Van Tinteren H, Graf N, Bergeron C, Sandstedt B, de Kraker J. Treatment of pulmonary metastases in children with stage IV nephroblastoma with risk-based use of pulmonary radiotherapy. Journal of Clinical Oncology: Official Journal of the

American Society of Clinical Oncology. 2012;**30**(28):3533-3539

[28] Dix DB, Seibel NL, Chi YY, Khanna G, Gratias E, Anderson JR, et al. Treatment of stage IV favorable histology wilms tumor with lung metastases: A report from the children's oncology group AREN0533 study. Journal of Clinical Oncology. 2018;**36**(16):1564-1570

[29] Mulder RL, Hudson MM, Bhatia S, Landier W, Levitt G, Constine LS, et al. Updated breast cancer surveillance recommendations for female survivors of childhood, adolescent, and Young adult cancer from the international guideline harmonization group. Journal of Clinical Oncology : Official Journal of the American Society of Clinical Oncology. 2020;**38**(35):4194-4207

[30] Spreafico F, Fernandez CV, Brok J, Nakata K, Vujanic G, Geller JI, et al. Wilms tumour. Nat Rev Dis Primers. 2021;**7**(1):75

[31] Perrone L, Sinisi AA, Sicuranza R, Di Tullio MT, Indolfi P, Giuliano MG, et al. Prepubertal endocrine follow-up in subjects with Wilms' tumor. Medical and Pediatric Oncology. 1988;**16**(4):255-258

[32] Shalet SM, Beardwell CG, Jacobs HS, Pearson D. Testicular function following irradiation of the human prepubertal testis. Clinical Endocrinology. 1978;**9**(6):483-490

[33] Green DM, Lange JM, Peabody EM, Grigorieva NN, Peterson SM, Kalapurakal JA, et al. Pregnancy outcome after treatment for Wilms tumor: A report from the national Wilms tumor long-term follow-up study. Journal of Clinical Oncology. 2010;**28**(17):2824-2830

[34] Nussbaum Blask AR, Nicholson HS, Markle BM, Wechsler-Jentzch K, O'Donnell R, Byrne J. Sonographic detection of uterine and ovarian abnormalities in female survivors of Wilms' tumor treated with radiotherapy. AJR. American Journal of Roentgenology. 1999;**172**(3):759-763

[35] Li FP, Gimbrere K, Gelber RD, Sallan SE, Flamant F, Green DM, et al. Outcome of pregnancy in survivors of Wilms' tumor. Journal of the American Medical Association. 1987;**257**(2):216-219

[36] Byrne J, Mulvihill JJ, Connelly RR, Austin DA, Holmes GE, Holmes FF, et al. Reproductive problems and birth defects in survivors of Wilms' tumor and their relatives. Medical and Pediatric Oncology. 1988;**16**(4):233-240

[37] Green DM, Peabody EM, Nan B, Peterson S, Kalapurakal JA, Breslow NE. Pregnancy outcome after treatment for Wilms tumor: A report from the National Wilms Tumor Study Group. Journal of Clinical Oncology. 2002;**20**(10):2506-2513

[38] Kalapurakal JA, Peterson S, Peabody EM, Thomas PR, Green DM, D'Angio GJ, et al. Pregnancy outcomes after abdominal irradiation that included or excluded the pelvis in childhood Wilms tumor survivors: A report from the National Wilms Tumor Study. International Journal of Radiation Oncology, Biology, Physics. 2004;**58**(5):1364-1368

[39] van der Perk MEM, Cost NG, Bos AME, Brannigan R, Chowdhury T, Davidoff AM, et al. White paper: Onco-fertility in pediatric patients with Wilms tumor. International Journal of Cancer. 2022;**151**(6):843-858

[40] Mulder RL, Font-Gonzalez A, Hudson MM, van Santen HM, Loeffen EAH, Burns KC, et al. Fertility preservation for female patients with

childhood, adolescent, and young adult cancer: Recommendations from the PanCareLIFE consortium and the international late effects of childhood cancer guideline harmonization group. The Lancet Oncology. 2021;**22**(2):e45-e56

[41] Green DM, Lange JM, Qu A, Peterson SM, Kalapurakal JA, Stokes DC, et al. Pulmonary disease after treatment for Wilms tumor: A report from the national Wilms tumor long-term follow-up study. Pediatric Blood & Cancer. 2013;**60**(10):1721-1726

[42] Foster KL, Salehabadi SM, Green DM, Xing M, Ness KK, Krull KR, et al. Clinical assessment of late health outcomes in survivors of Wilms tumor. Pediatrics. 2022;**150**(5):e2022056918

[43] Wallace WH, Shalet SM, Morris-Jones PH, Swindell R, Gattamaneni HR. Effect of abdominal irradiation on growth in boys treated for a Wilms' tumor. Medical and Pediatric Oncology. 1990;**18**(6):441-446

[44] Probert JC, Parker BR, Kaplan HS. Growth retardation in children after megavoltage irradiation of the spine. Cancer. 1973;**32**(3):634-639

[45] Rubin P, Duthie RB, Young LW. The significance of scoliosis in postirradiated Wilms's tumor and neuroblastoma. Radiology. 1962;**79**:539-559

[46] Thomas PR, Griffith KD, Fineberg BB, Perez CA, Land VJ. Late effects of treatment for Wilms' tumor. International Journal of Radiation Oncology, Biology, Physics. 1983;**9**(5):651-657

[47] Oliver JH, Gluck G, Gledhill RB, Chevalier L. Musculoskeletal deformities following treatment of Wilms' tumour. Canadian Medical Association Journal. 1978;**119**(5):459-464

[48] Mäkipernaa A, Heikkilä JT, Merikanto J, Marttinen E, Siimes MA. Spinal deformity induced by radiotherapy for solid tumours in childhood: A long-term follow up study. European Journal of Pediatrics. 1993;**152**(3):197-200

[49] Silverman CL, Thomas PR, McAlister WH, Walker S, Whiteside LA. Slipped femoral capital epiphyses in irradiated children: Dose, volume and age relationships. International Journal of Radiation Oncology, Biology, Physics. 1981;7(10):1357-1363

[50] Interiano RB, Delos Santos N, Huang S, Srivastava DK, Robison LL, Hudson MM, et al. Renal function in survivors of nonsyndromic Wilms tumor treated with unilateral radical nephrectomy. Cancer. 2015;**121**(14):2449-2456

[51] de Graaf SS, van Gent H, Reitsma-Bierens WC, van Luyk WH, Dolsma WV, Postma A. Renal function after unilateral nephrectomy for Wilms' tumour: The influence of radiation therapy. European Journal of Cancer. 1996;**32A**(3):465-469

[52] Bárdi E, Oláh AV, Bartyik K, Endreffy E, Jenei C, Kappelmayer J, et al. Late effects on renal glomerular and tubular function in childhood cancer survivors. Pediatric Blood & Cancer. 2004;**43**(6):668-673

[53] Breslow NE, Collins AJ, Ritchey ML, Grigoriev YA, Peterson SM, Green DM. End stage renal disease in patients with Wilms tumor: Results from the National Wilms Tumor Study Group and the United States renal data system. The Journal of Urology. 2005;**174**(5):1972-1975

[54] Lange J, Peterson SM, Takashima JR, Grigoriev Y, Ritchey ML,

Shamberger RC, et al. Risk factors for end stage renal disease in non-WT1-syndromic Wilms tumor. The Journal of Urology. 2011;**186**(2):378-386

[55] Hogsholt S, Asdahl PH, Rechnitzer C, Winther JF, Birn H, Hasle H. Kidney disease in very long-term survivors of Wilms tumor: A nationwide cohort study with sibling controls. Cancer Medicine. 2022;**12**(2):1330-1338

[56] Dekkers IA, Blijdorp K, Cransberg K, Pluijm SM, Pieters R, Neggers SJ, et al. Long-term nephrotoxicity in adult survivors of childhood cancer. Clinical Journal of the American Society of Nephrology. 2013;**8**(6):922-929

[57] Teinturier C, Tournade MF, Caillat-Zucman S, Boitard C, Amoura Z, Bougneres PF, et al. Diabetes mellitus after abdominal radiation therapy. Lancet. 1995;**346**(8975):633-634

[58] Holmqvist AS, Olsen JH, Andersen KK, de Fine LS, Hjorth L, Garwicz S, et al. Adult life after childhood cancer in Scandinavia: Diabetes mellitus following treatment for cancer in childhood. European Journal of Cancer. 2014;**50**(6):1169-1175

[59] Friedman DN, Moskowitz CS, Hilden P, Howell RM, Weathers RE, Smith SA, et al. Radiation dose and volume to the pancreas and subsequent risk of diabetes mellitus: A report from the childhood cancer survivor study. Journal of the National Cancer Institute. 2020;**112**(5):525-532

[60] Kalapurakal JA, Gopalakrishnan M, Mille M, Helenowski I, Peterson S, Rigsby C, et al. Feasibility and accuracy of UF/NCI phantoms and Monte Carlo retrospective dosimetry in children treated on National Wilms Tumor Study protocols. Pediatric Blood & Cancer. 2018;**65**(12):e27395

[61] Robison LL, Armstrong GT, Boice JD, Chow EJ, Davies SM, Donaldson SS, et al. The childhood cancer survivor study: A National Cancer Institute-supported resource for outcome and intervention research. Journal of Clinical Oncology. 2009;**27**(14):2308-2318

[62] Lange JM, Takashima JR, Peterson SM, Kalapurakal JA, Green DM, Breslow NE. Breast cancer in female survivors of Wilms tumor: A report from the national Wilms tumor late effects study. Cancer. 2014;**120**(23):3722-3730

[63] Bhayana S, Song F, Jacob J, Fadda P, Denko NC, Xu-Welliver M, et al. Urinary miRNAs as biomarkers for noninvasive evaluation of radiation-induced renal tubular injury. Radiation Research. 2017;**188**(6):626-635

[64] Inker LA, Wyatt C, Creamer R, Hellinger J, Hotta M, Leppo M, et al. Performance of creatinine and cystatin C GFR estimating equations in an HIV-positive population on antiretrovirals. Journal of Acquired Immune Deficiency Syndromes. 2012;**61**(3):302-309

[65] Kim Y, Seidman JG, Seidman CE. Genetics of cancer therapy-associated cardiotoxicity. Journal of Molecular and Cellular Cardiology. 2022;**167**:85-91

[66] Morton LM, Sampson JN, Armstrong GT, Chen TH, Hudson MM, Karlins E, et al. Genome-wide association study to identify susceptibility loci that modify radiation-related risk for breast cancer after childhood cancer. Journal of the National Cancer Institute. 2017;**109**(11):djx058

[67] Brooke RJ, Im C, Wilson CL, Krasin MJ, Liu Q, Li Z, et al. A high-risk haplotype for premature menopause in childhood cancer survivors exposed to Gonadotoxic therapy. Journal of the National Cancer Institute. 2018;**110**(8):895-904

[68] Kline RM, Arora NK, Bradley CJ, Brauer ER, Graves DL, Lunsford NB, et al. Long-term survivorship care after cancer treatment—Summary of a 2017 National Cancer Policy Forum Workshop. Journal of the National Cancer Institute. 2018;**110**(12):1300-1310

[69] Horowitz ME, Fordis M, Krause S, McKellar J, Poplack DG. Passport for care: Implementing the survivorship care plan. Journal of Oncology Practice/ American Society of Clinical Oncology. 2009;**5**(3):110-112

[70] Eshelman-Kent D, Kinahan KE, Hobbie W, Landier W, Teal S, Friedman D, et al. Cancer survivorship practices, services, and delivery: A report from the Children's oncology group (COG) nursing discipline, adolescent/young adult, and late effects committees. Journal of Cancer Survivorship. 2011;**5**(4):345-357

[71] Nathan PC, Ford JS, Henderson TO, Hudson MM, Emmons KM, Casillas JN, et al. Health behaviors, medical care, and interventions to promote healthy living in the childhood cancer survivor study cohort. Journal of Clinical Oncology. 2009;**27**(14):2363-2373

[72] Nathan PC, Daugherty CK, Wroblewski KE, Kigin ML, Stewart TV, Hlubocky FJ, et al. Family physician preferences and knowledge gaps regarding the care of adolescent and young adult survivors of childhood cancer. Journal of Cancer Survivorship. 2013;**7**(3):275-282

[73] Cox CL, Zhu L, Ojha RP, Li C, Srivastava DK, Riley BB, et al. The unmet emotional, care/support, and informational needs of adult survivors of pediatric malignancies. Journal of Cancer Survivorship. 2016;**10**(4):743-758

[74] McAleer MF, Melchior P, Parkes J, Pater L, Rube C, Saunders D, et al. Harmonica consensus, controversies, and future directions in radiotherapy for pediatric Wilms tumors. Pediatric Blood & Cancer. 2022:e30090